THE MEANING OF BEHAVIORS IN DEMENTIA/NEURCOGNITIVE DISORDERS: NEW TERMINOLOGY, CLASSIFICATION, AND BEHAVIORAL MANAGEMENT

WRITTEN BY
ATUL SUNNY LUTHRA

EDITED BY
JAMES BOURGEOIS

THE MEANING OF BEHAVIORS IN DEMENTIA/NEURCOGNITIVE DISORDERS: NEW TERMINOLOGY, CLASSIFICATION, AND BEHAVIORAL MANAGEMENT

WRITTEN BY
ATUL SUNNY LUTHRA

EDITED BY
JAMES BOURGEOIS

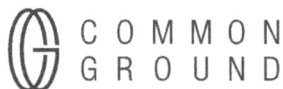

COMMON GROUND

First published in 2014 in Champaign, Illinois, USA
by Common Ground Publishing LLC
as part of the Aging in Society book series

Library of Congress Cataloging-in-Publication Data

Luthra, Atul Sunny, 1962- author.
  The meaning of behaviors in dementia/neurocognitive disorders : new terminology, classification,
and behavioral management / Atul Sunny Luthra.
      p. ; cm. -- (Aging in society)
  Includes bibliographical references.
  ISBN 978-1-61229-532-9 (pbk : alk. paper) -- ISBN 978-1-61229-533-6 (pdf)
  I. Title. II. Series: Aging in society (Series)
  [DNLM: 1. Dementia--classification. 2. Behavioral Symptoms. 3. Cognition Disorders--
classification. 4. Cognition Disorders--diagnosis. 5. Dementia--diagnosis. 6. Terminology as
Topic. WM 15]

  RC394.C64
  616.8'3--dc23

                              2014021521

Cover image photo credit: Phillip Kalantzis-Cope

Table of Contents

Acknowledgements

This book is dedicated to Kenneth Murray, founder of the Murray Alzheimer's Research and Educational Program (MAREP), at University of Waterloo. Mr. Murray has demonstrated himself to be a visionary in the area of dementia/NCD care in Canada and around the world. I would like to thank Heather Foster, MAREP student in 2009-10, and Kathleen Dobson, MAREP student in 2012-13, for reviewing the literature on these constructs and in helping to write the initial drafts of this book. Finally, I would like to thank Trevor Semplonius, MAREP student in 2011-12, for helping me write the final version of the chapters. Trevor has stayed with me as a research assistant and has provided continued support with formatting and finalizing the bibliography for this book. Trevor has been a constant support for me in this and several other research projects. I would like to thank Dr. Bourgeois for agreeing to assist me in editing and formatting this book, thereby making it an invaluable source of information for all health care professionals working in the field of Dementia/NCD care.

Editorial Note

In order to conform to DSM-5 language, wherein the familiar term "dementia" has been supplanted by "major/mild neurocognitive disorder (NCD)", this volume will use the term "dementia/NCD" throughout the text, except in direct quotations and reference citations.

Chapter 1: Preface

With moderate stage dementia/NCD, he was removed by several degrees from reality. Approaching a co-patient, he proceeded to throw his beverage upon him. It was witnessed. Staff intervened, controlling the situation. This unassuming elderly man had triggered a cascade of events. What followed was not unusual; similar efforts were undertaken when involving other patients. Discourse amongst staff ensued to attempt to ascertain the meaning for the seemingly "unprovoked aggression". This gentleman spoke only French his primary language, his previous mastery in English having eroded. Believing that his residence was a chapel and unable to identify cues he was residing in a long term care (LTC) facility, he misidentified his role as being the janitor, his life's occupation. He spent most of the day wandering the LTC unit, "lost" in his own singular reality. Amnestic, the meaning behind his aggressive actions could not be captured in his testimony. It was left to clinicians to wade through the mire of confusion and navigate a plan and safe outcome by attempting to understand his reality unveiling the *meaning* inherent in his behavior.

Many varied and hypothetical meanings potentially underlying the aggression were placed forth, all plausible. They spanned the biological, (was he medically unwell?); psychological, (was he missing his wife, sad or depressed?) and social, (did he believe the co-patient an intruder in his "chapel'" thus attempt to protect himself from the '"trespasser"?) Equally valid perceptions, but staff found themselves again without a means to clarify. For clinicians lacked a comprehensive, comprehensible and concise tool to assess the presenting behavior whereby the findings would be consistent and assist in formulating a treatment plan. This was not atypical. On the contrary rather typical, depicting the current ubiquitous landscape in management of patients exhibiting behavioral and psychological symptoms of dementia/NCD (BPSD) in LTC.

The prevalence of dementia/NCD will increase proportional to the increase number of aged in North America and the rest of the developed world over the upcoming decades, an inverse population pyramid representing this demographic trend. "Seniors make up the fastest-growing age group. This trend is expected to continue for the next several decades. In 2011 an estimated 5.0 million Canadians were 65 years of age or older, a number that is expected to double in the next 25 years, reach[ing] 10.4 million seniors by 2036." (Human Resources and Skills Development Canada, 2013). Compounding matters further, the now infamous

2010 Alzheimer's Society *Rising Tide* report estimates that" in 2038 the incidence of dementia will increase to one new case diagnosed every two minutes, equal to 257, 800 Canadian cases per year" (World Health Organization, 2012). The weight of this is abysmal. These trends are impacting the direct and indirect costs associated with dementia/NCD care; both are rising proportionately (World Health Organization, 2012).

According to ICD-10's Clinical Descriptions and Diagnostic Guidelines for Mental and Behavioral Disorders, dementia/NCD is defined as "a decline in memory, which is most evident in the learning of new information, although in more severe cases, the recall of previously learned information may be also affected. The impairment applies to both verbal and non-verbal material. The decline should be objectively verified by obtaining a reliable history from an informant, supplemented, if possible, by neuropsychological tests or quantified cognitive assessments" (Wetterling et al., 1994). The guidelines further describe three consecutive stages in dementia/NCD whereby patients transition through mild, moderate, and severe [or advanced].

In the early stages of care of patients with dementia/NCD, the focus is on evaluation of cognitive decline and its impact on functional deficits and associated risks. One of the primary reasons for this emphasis is the availability of pharmacological treatments in the form of cholinesterase inhibitors (Liperoti et al., 2008). Additionally, clinicians have at their disposal cognitive assessment evidence based tools with sound clinical utility such as the Mini Mental State Examination (MMSE) © (Folstein, M.F., Folstein, S.E. & McHugh, P.R., 1975) not to mention a host of others. These are enmeshed in the fabric of assessment for dementia/NCD; so much so, that the Ontario Drug Benefit funding for pharmacological cognitive enhancement treatment is contingent upon the MMSE© test score (Ontario Ministry of Health and Long-term Care, 2005).

As the illness progresses to the moderate and advanced stages, however, the development of behavioral and psychological symptoms in dementia/NCD (BPSD) are increasingly more common, eventually becoming prevalent in over 90% of cases (Liperoti et al., 2008). Also known as responsive behaviors, BPSD refers to the non-cognitive neuropsychiatric symptoms of "disturbed perceptions, thought content, and mood or behavior that frequently occur in patients with dementia/NCD" (Finkel and Burns, 1999). The spectrum of behaviors may include aggression, agitation and restlessness, anxiety, pacing, screaming, depression, psychosis, sleep disturbance, shadowing, "sundowning" (agitation in the evening/overnight), wandering, hoarding, cursing, swearing, repetitive vocalization, pacing and repetitive motor activity (Scottish Intercollegiate Guidelines Network, 2006).

Not surprisingly BPSD profoundly negatively affects the quality of life of dementia/NCD patients and their families alike (Black & Almeida, 2004). The presence of BPSD has been shown to have a deleterious impact on caregiver stress, admission to LTC facilities, problematic adjustment to a LTC environment, morbidity, and even mortality (Black & Almeida, 2004). Acknowledging this, the 2012 report on dementia/NCD issued by the World Health Organization recognized the need for [equally] effective treatment of behavioral symptoms [as is the case for cognitive symptoms] as a necessary goal for improving outcomes in dementia/NCD care (World Health Organization, 2012).

Patients entering LTC homes are older in the current environment. Consequently, they are more likely to suffer from dementia/NCD and its neuropsychiatric sequelae, BPSD. "According to an extensive investigation into abuse at Canadian LTC homes by Canadian Television Network (a private broadcasting network based in Ontario, Canada), there were at least 6,500 documented cases of resident-on-resident attacks in 2012, [residents being synonymous with patients]" (CARP action on Nursing Home Violence, 2013). Lamented as a tragedy, the injurious outcomes of BPSD exhibited by residents in LTC have yet to reach an apex. Groups are speaking out and calling for change. The Ontario Association of Non-Profit Homes and Services for seniors in there 2005 Position paper advocated for "better assessment tools, more coordinated services, more resources to support creative models within communities and increased funding to support the needs of those with complex mental health issues" (Alzheimer Society, 2005). Of the 85 recommendations stemming from the 2005 Coroner inquest into the 2001 Casa Verde Case- a harrowing LTC patient-on-patient assault ending gravely. The assaulted patient ended up succumbing to his injuries. - "the need for better communication and comprehensive assessments were noted as consistent messages heard before" (Alzheimer Society, 2005) and the same rings true today. Engaging this concern, in 2011 the Ministry of Health and Long Term Care invested $40 million in Behavioral Supports Ontario to train and provide quality care to these residents [or patients] (Alzheimer Knowledge Exchange Resource Centre, 2013).

Favorable progress yes, but this is not a complete panacea. For therein lays a broad reach of uncertainty magnified by a lack of confidence in available assessment tools and scant approved pharmacological treatment options for behaviors related to moderate and advanced stage dementia/NCD. Indeed literature consistently demonstrates a relative paucity of reliable and valid assessment scales for patients with moderate to advanced stages of dementia/NCD (Morandi et al., 2012).

Without exception, as was the situation with our French-speaking gentelman, with diagnosis of BPSD, in accordance with DSM criteria is one of exclusion. All major mood, anxiety, psychotic spectrum disorders and delirium require ruling out prior to symptoms being diagnosed BPSD. This is practicable in the early stages of dementia/NCD. Here it is possible to obtain a history from the patient and conduct a formal mental status examination with an appropriate physical examination, distinguishing amongst different clinical states ruling out psychiatric co-morbid illness, using established DSM-5 criteria. Herein lays the challenge. With progression of cognitive impairment through moderate to advanced, there is decreased reliability and validity of the history and mental status exam conducted. Under such conditions, greater emphasis is placed upon obtaining collateral information from alternate sources and on clinical observations, more so than clinical interview of the patient. Thus, the diagnosis of specific clinical states psychiatric co-morbidity or distinguishing amongst clinical states, in accordance with DSM is increasingly difficult and challenging (World Health Organization, 2012).

Moreover, when BPSD is diagnosed, evidence for effective pharmacological treatment is not convincing. The equivocal evidence of benefits and deleterious effects from atypical antipsychotics for this indication tends to discourage their use or leads to them being used sparingly (Seitz et al., 2013). Although limited, much of the available evidence seems to suggest increased morbidity from the use of atypical antipsychotics in the absence of robust benefits [for this cohort] (Seitz et al., 2013). Likewise, evidence for use of other classes of psychotropic medications (e.g., mood stabilizers, antidepressants, and benzodiazepines) is also equivocal (Seitz et al., 2013). Lack of evidence for use of all classes of psychotropic medications in the management of BPSD and high risks of morbidity and mortality from their use has resulted in guidelines proposing minimal prescribing of these medications. In 2005 the U.S. FDA issued a "black box" warning reporting a 1.6 time increased risk of death for persons with Alzheimer's dementia/NCD receiving atypical agents (Madhusoodanan et al., 2007). In Canada, risperidone is the only antipsychotic approved for this indication.

Accordingly, best practice guidelines in treatment of BPSD are generated based in the first principle of practice of medicine: *primum non nocere* (do no harm). Subsequently, non-pharmacological interventions, both interpersonal and environmental, are proposed as first line in management of behaviors in all stages of dementia/NCD. The majority of evidence for non-pharmacological interventions comes from observational and case-based studies. These tend to demonstrate only modest benefits (Livingston et al., 2005). Although there are a few randomized control trials, major limitations exist in demonstrating efficacy of non-pharmacological interventions in managing behaviors in patients with dementia/NCD (Teri et al., 2003; Chenoweth et al., 2009). Even then, when these interventions are proven effective as Corbett et al. (2012) state, "despite positive outcomes, it can be difficult to implement these individualized interventions in all settings due to the level of skill required among care staff". Furthermore, the high and unsustainable economic cost of these interventions is a limiting consideration (Corbett et al., 2012). Currently, the cost of managing BPSD accounts for over 30% of the total annual cost of dementia/NCD care and is projected to increase exponentially, mirroring the projected prevalence trends of dementia/NCD (Schnaider Beeri et al., 2002; World Health Organization, 2012).

It is concerning for behavioral management in dementia/NCD care, with such far reaching multifaceted implications, to have so few pharmacological treatment options and such expensive and unsustainable non-pharmacological treatments available to lessen the burden.

As a way forward, the recent literature encourages health care professionals to find "meaning" for the presence of behaviors in patients with dementia/NCD, towards advancing both pharmacological and non-pharmacological treatments. "Meaning" refers to understanding the reasons for the presence of behaviors from the patient's point of view, (e.g. what is the patient attempting to express or communicate in the absence of their ability to communicate through language? as is often the case in moderate to advance stage dementia/NCD and when the presence of behaviors is highest.)

Tragically, there is a paucity of literature and assessment tools to provide guidance in determining "meaning". The PIECES model of dementia/NCD care provides a best practice, systematic approach to enhancing the care of the older person with complex physical, cognitive and mental health needs (Hamilton, Harris & Le Clair, 2006). It provides an approach to the understanding of the presence of behaviors in this patient population and for development of safe interventions. The model utilizes a comprehensive, interdisciplinary person-centered approach to assessment and intervention for the behavioral risks. The initial three letter **P-I-E** stand for **P**hysical, **I**ntellectual and **E**motional health of the patient. The **C** stands for **C**apabilities the drive to maximize them in order to achieve the best quality of life for the patient. The **E-S** stands for the **E**nvironment in which the patient lives and **S** stands for the **S**ocial Self of the patient (cultural and spiritual life history). This model of care approaches behaviors as a way of identifying various antecedents which may be contributory to behavioral occurrences (Hamilton, Harris & Le Clair, 2006). The PIECES model lacks direction on understanding the "meaning" of behaviors which often persist despite addressing all contributing factors. The Gentle Persuasive Approach (GPA) to dementia care is also based in principles of person centered care (Speziale et al., 2009). Front line staff are taught approaches which empower them to respond effectively, and with respect, to the needs of dementia patients which are often expressed through responsive behaviors (Speziale et al., 2009). Managing behaviors does allude to making all efforts at understanding the "meaning" of behaviors in dementia/NCD. GPA encourages the understanding of behaviors in the context of "personhood" of the patient (Speziale et al., 2009). However, it does not provide any specific construct which can be applied to presenting behaviors to understand what they are meaning or expressing from the patient's point of view. Thus, despite established consensus around the need to understand the "meaning" of behaviors as a way to better manage patients, there exists a relative paucity of paradigms, tools or constructs afforded clinicians to do so.

Further complicating finding the "meaning" is the absence of a biopsychosocial (BPS) model for understanding the reasons for occurrence of behaviors in dementia/NCD. Absence of such seriously limits the ability of any existing model to be used as a valid classification system for behaviors in dementia/NCD. Presently, all existing models for understanding the "meaning" of occurrence of behaviors are dichotomized along either biological or psychosocial paradigms only. BPSD terminology is not currently supported by any existing model combining BPS variables for their presence.

In addition, once BPSD is diagnosed, no classification system exists to further breakdown the behavioral symptoms into meaningful clusters. Even the most fundamentally rudimentary constructs for defining reference terminology and classification systems have yet to be developed in the area of behaviors in dementia/NCD. This chasm requires bridging for any substantive progress to occur in either assessment or treatment. Hence, we first need to both understand and value the way patients with dementia/NCD view the world uncovering concerns from that lens towards development of a classification system thereby facilitating efficacious assessment and treatment.

In the absence of valid measures to accurately diagnose behavioral symptoms in moderate to advanced stage dementia/NCD, it is challenging to aggregate them into clinically meaningful categories. These behavioral symptoms have yet to be grouped into clusters, which are either consistent along temporal lines or respond to a common pharmacological treatment; the primary criteria requiring fulfillment in order to diagnose syndromes.

Proposed Classification Model for BPSD

Literature identifies biological, personal (psychological) and environmental (social) variables contributory to the occurrence of behaviors in dementia/NCD. The author reviewed each at length forming the premise in development of a new dynamic model of interactions towards understanding the meaning for the presence of behaviors in patients with dementia/NCD. Incorporating a BPS model and applying reference terminology to behaviors in dementia/NCD, the author has developed a novel classification system for use in assessment of behaviors in patients with moderate to advanced stage dementia/NCD.

   Reference terminology is defined as "a set of concepts and relationships that provide a common reference point for comparisons and aggregation of data" (Imel & Campbell, 2003). A *classification system* is defined as "a systematic arrangement into classes or groups based on perceived common characteristics; a means of giving order to a group of disconnected facts. The groups or classes may have similar or like characteristics or may even be synonymous" (Imel & Campbell, 2003). When these definitions are applied to the area of behaviors in dementia/NCDs, "terminology" begins with identification and incorporation of all variables which are contributory to the generation of behaviors. Only once all these variables are incorporated into a BPS model defining intricate relationships amongst them to "provide a common reference point" can any classification begin. It is this "common reference point" that is used to propose a new classification system applicable to behaviors in moderate to advanced stage dementia/NCD.

   Derived from synthesizing existing constructs in developmental and behavioral psychology in addition to dementia/NCD literature, each behavioral category or domain represents a collection of "alike" or "similar" behavioral symptoms which (Davis, et al.1997)

   1. Adequately represent the category/domain
   2. Provide 'meaning' or 'purpose' for the existence of the category/domain,
   3. Provides that of each category/domain can be adequately justified by specific theoretical constructs or principles derived from existing literature.

Chapter Outline

Chapter 2 provides a historical overview of the existing terminologies and models recognizing limitations associated with them thus serving as a springboard for the model development. In Chapter 3 a biopsychosocial model for understanding the occurrence of behaviors in moderate to late stage dementia/NCD is introduced. Labeled stage congruent responsive behaviors (SCRB), this proposed model, based upon principals identified by Davis et al., forms the foundation for the new behavioral classification system. Chapter three further elaborates on the SCRB model forming the foundation additionally for the justification of new terminology for behaviors in dementia/NCD.

Throughout Chapters 4 to 8, literature reviewed is examined identifying the specification of the theoretical construct for aggregation of similar behavioral symptoms into clinically meaningful categories using the SCRB model. Means to assess for these behavioral symptoms and proposed approaches in managing their presentation is reviewed for each.

To elaborate further, in chapter 4, the author examines those behavioral categories based in theories on information processing. Two behavioral categories emanating from pathological changes in theories of information processing are disorganized behaviors and misidentification behaviors. In chapter 5 behavioral constructs identified are based upon motivational and needs based theories. Behavioral categories emanating from these two constructs are apathy behaviors, goal directed behaviors, motor behaviors and importuning behaviors. Chapter 6 examines constructs for behavioral categories in theories on regulation of emotions. Behavioral categories emanating from this construct are emotional behaviors, fretful/trepidated behaviors and vocal behaviors. Behavioral category theories on compliance and aggression are examined in chapter 7. From here oppositional behaviors and physically aggressive behavior categories flow. The final behavioral category stems from all of theories in information processing, motivational and needs based theories, theories in regulation of emotions and self-stimulatory theories combined. The two behavioral categories emanating from these constructs are vocal behaviors and sexual behaviors are discussed in chapter 8. Chapter 9 provides a summary of all the proposed constructs as well as future direction with this paradigm is outlined, in research and clinical settings.

This book provides understanding for the reasons surrounding the present state of practice in behavioral assessment and treatment of moderate to advanced stage dementia/NCD, justifying the approach in the development of a novel classification and labeling system. As a teaching tool and clinical reference manual this book will educate clinicians on applying this new classification to behaviors in dementia/NCD improving practice and patient outcomes.

It is the author's hope that this novel classification system will inform clinicians understanding of the "meaning" of behaviors when patient observations are of paramount importance in assessment. It is further envisaged improving quality of life through informed assessment towards efficacious treatment will be realized. Finally, optimizing care delivery costs for this population such as with our French-speaking gentleman and so many others to follow is paramount.

In this paradox, patients and clinicians alike wander the terrain of behaviors in dementia/NCD assembled towards a common goal, meaning. Where patients struggle to divulge that meaning which is camouflaged, clinicians seek to understand the meaning that they challenged to discern. Yet, "not all who wander are lost" (Tolkien, 1954). Let this be the posture we aspire to in behavioral assessment of persons with dementia/NCD. For who will continue to be truly lost and wandering seeking meaning remains in question. *Ensemble, dans la poursuite de sens.* (Together in the pursuit of meaning.)

Chapter 2: Evolution of Concepts in Terminology

The terminology used to label and describe the non-cognitive or behavioral symptoms of dementia/NCD has evolved from disruptive, agitation, and aggression, to the umbrella term "Behavioral and Psychological Symptoms of Dementia/NCD"; referred to as "BPSD" (Smith & Buckwalter, 2005) and "Responsive Behaviors" (Dupuis et al., 2004).

Disruptive, Disturbing & Problem Behaviors in Dementia/NCD

The terms "disruptive," "disturbing," and "problem" are amongst the earliest terms used in dementia/NCD care to broadly label behaviors in dementia/NCD (Smith & Buckwalter, 2005). Vague interpretations were drawn based on the meaning of these terms which aim to cover a range of disparate symptoms. In addition, these terms tended to be a negative reflection of "the caregiver's view of the disease rather than the cognitively-impaired person's perspective in a given situation" (Algase et al., 1996; Smith and Buckwalter 2005).

Agitation in Dementia/NCD

Cohen-Mansfield and Billig (1986) developed a very specific definition of agitation in context of the dementia/NCD population. This definition describes agitation as the "inappropriate verbal, vocal, or motor activity that is not explained by needs or confusion *per s*e" (Cohen-Mansfield & Billig, 1986). Under these criteria, behaviors in dementia/NCD can be labeled as "agitation" only after mood, anxiety, and psychotic disorders, delirium, and unmet needs have been ruled out (Cohen-Mansfield, 2003). It is a very specific clinical construct and has a behavioral assessment scale developed on this principle for use in dementia/NCD, the *Cohen-Mansfield Agitation Inventory Scale* (Cohen-Mansfield & Billig, 1986; Cohen-Mansfield, 2003).

Aggression in Dementia/NCD

Definition of aggression in context of dementia/NCD was defined by Patel and Hope (1992) as, "an overt act, involving the delivery of noxious stimuli to (but not necessarily aimed at) another organism, object or self, which is clearly accidental". Aggressive behaviors have been identified to include physical aggression, aggressive resistance, physical threats, verbal aggression, refusing to speak, destructive behavior, and general irritability (Patel & Hope, 1992). Aggressive behaviors could also be defined to include physical, verbal, or sexual aggression (Patel & Hope, 1992); however, specific types of aggression are not always stipulated in published studies and it is used as an umbrella term. Furthermore, based upon Patel and Hope's (1992) definition, it is not clear if aggressive behavior within dementia/NCD is labeled after the occurrence of one act or if recurrent acts are required. To compound matters further, evidence has been presented that the perception of care providers as to which behaviors are considered to be aggressive, is a subjective and not always reliable statement (Pulsford & Duxbury, 2006).

Behavioral and Psychological Symptoms of Dementia/NCD (BPSD)

Behavioral and Psychological Symptoms of Dementia/NCD (BPSD) is an all-encompassing term established to label all non-cognitive symptoms of dementia/NCD (Smith & Buckwalter, 2005). It was defined by Smith and Buckwalter (2005) as, "agitation and aggression, apathy and withdrawal, anxiety, irritability, dysphoria and depression, disinhibition, delusions, hallucinations and paranoia, as well as including activities such as wandering, socially inappropriate behavior, and resistance to care." Diagnosis of BPSD, in accordance with DSM-5 criteria, does require mood, anxiety, psychotic spectrum disorders and delirium to be ruled out prior to symptoms being labeled as BPSD. Furthermore, all reversible medical conditions deemed to be contributory to presenting behaviors must be ruled out. BPSD is the most universal term used to describe non-cognitive characteristics of dementia/NCD and has been accepted by the International Psychogeriatric Association as well as incorporated into the DSM-5 (American Psychiatric Association, 2000).

Responsive Behaviors in Dementia/NCD

In the recent years, the term "responsive" has been used to label behaviors in dementia/NCD, instead of the terms described above (Dupuis et al., 2004). Dupuis et al. (2004) have proposed the following criteria to further the understanding of the term "responsive" behaviors:

- It reflects a response to something negative, frustrating or confusing in the person's environment
- The term "responsive" behaviors places the reasons for behaviors "outside" of the persons rather than "within" the individual ("within" referring to biological processes)

- Persons with dementia/NCD chose this term with the reasoning that behavior is a means of communicating;
- To address behaviors and need to change physical or social aspects environment

Limitations of Current Terminology

Diagnosis of BPSD, in accordance with DSM criteria, does require all major mood, anxiety and psychotic spectrum disorders to be ruled out prior to symptoms being labeled as BPSD. In the early stages of dementia/NCD when it is possible to obtain a history from the patient and conduct a formal mental status examination with an appropriate physical examination, diagnosis of psychiatric co-morbidity, using established DSM-5, criteria, can be achieved. The same can be achieved, when applying Cohen-Mansfield criteria, to identify agitation in patients with dementia/NCD. Diagnosing BPSD or *agitation* can only be done when a valid and a reliable clinical examination can be conducted, as is the case in early stages.

With advancing stages of cognitive impairment, there is decreased reliability and validity of the history and mental status exam conducted with the patient. Under these conditions, greater emphasis is placed upon obtaining collateral information from other sources and on clinical observations more so than clinical interview of the patient. Thus, the diagnosis of specific clinical states or distinguishing amongst clinical states, in accordance with DSM, is increasingly difficult and challenging with decreasing reliability and validity in patients with advanced stages of dementia or in patients with primary language abnormalities in context of cognitive impairment (World Health Organization, 2012).

Under these circumstances, terminology such as problem behaviors, disruptive behaviors, disturbing behaviors, behavioral problems, and agitation have all been cross-referenced when describing behaviors in dementia/NCD, in both clinical and research settings (Cohen-Mansfield & Billig, 1986). The terms disruptive and dysfunctional behaviors were used interchangeably within clinical and research settings despite the absence of a universal and concrete definition for either (Ballard et al., 1999). Numerous researchers have used the term agitation and aggression interchangeably; when describing the behavioral disturbances in dementia/NCDs. As is evident from the above discussion, various terminologies have been used to label and describe behaviors in moderate to advanced dementia/NCD Consequently, classification of these has been problematic due to different terminology utilized for describing the same symptoms and the same terms used with different meanings by different researchers (Ballard, Gray & Ayre, 1999; p.44).

BPSD is an inventory of a wide variety of disparate symptoms occurring in the course of a patient's journey with the disease of dementia/NCD. The term BPSD begins in the absence of a biopsychosocial model for understanding the occurrences of behaviors in patients with dementia/NCD; the absence of a "common reference point". Its definitions are all-encompassing and can only alert the health care professional to the vast heterogeneity of the nature and type symptoms that can be present in a patient with dementia/NCD. Furthermore, it does not define anything which is specific or elusive to moderate to advanced stages of dementia/NCD. Building a consensus on clinical relevance of individual symptoms, persistence of symptoms and definitions of terminology can often be difficult.

Although BPSD is a "gold standard" for use in clinical practice, it lacks precision, validity, and reliability for identification of specific syndromes in patients with moderate to advanced stages of dementia/NCD (McShane, 2000). As a consequence, it becomes rather challenging to evaluate the effect of pharmacological and non-pharmacological interventions in a systematic manner; as has been demonstrated by all randomized clinical trials on the evaluation of these interventions in this patient population.

In the absence of identification of valid and reliable behavioral syndromes in moderate to advanced stages of dementia/NCD, federal regulatory bodies in the USA, Canada, and the rest of the developed worldno longer approve medications to treat the diagnosis of BPSD per se. Thus far, *risperidone* is the only medication to be approved by FDA (USA) as an indication for treatment of BPSD. Regulatory bodies are insisting upon more precise terminology, better definitions of syndromes with increased validity and reliability of data before they will consider approval of medications for this indication. The DSM-IV-TR defines agitation as, "excessive motor activity associated with a feeling of inner tension" (American Psychiatric Association, 2000). Similarly, the Comprehensive Textbook of Psychiatry identifies agitation as, "severe anxiety associated with motor restlessness" (Kaplan & Sadock, 1995). Both of these broadly defined terms are based on description of psychiatric disorders in general psychiatry and are not specific towards dementia/NCD. Cohen-Mansfield (1986) did define a very specific clinical construct of agitation in context of dementia/NCD and which produces a very pure and a homogenous sample of agitation. "Agitation" in context of BPSD, is based on the definitions of Kaplan and Sadock (1995) and DSM-IV-TR (2000), and not Cohen-Mansfield (2003). The incidence of behaviors determined by current definition of BPSD, which uses the definition of agitation put forth by Kaplan and Sadock (1995) and DSM-IV-TR (2000), is present in upwards of 90% in dementia/NCD population (Cohen-Mansfield, 2003).

As per existing definitions, there is an inherent disconnect between the paradigm used to *label* behaviors and the one used to *quantify* behaviors. It is the definition put forth by Kaplan and Sadock (1995) and DSM-IV-TR which is being used, as a part of definition of BPSD, in clinical practice to label agitation behaviors. But it is *Cohen-Mansfield Agitation Inventory* (CMAI) that is utilized to quantify the frequency and severity of the identified behaviors (Morandi et al., 2012). This represents the current inadequate state of practice in the area of behaviors in dementia/NCD.

Standardized scales exist to help in distinguishing amongst various clinical conditions, albeit not BPSD per se, in dementia/NCD patients presenting with behaviors. This step is necessary, as the diagnosis of BPSD is one of exclusion. Examples of these scales include the *Cornell Scale for Depression in Dementia/NCD* and *Dementia/NCD Mood Assessment Scale*. These two scales are utilized to assess depression in dementia/NCD; however, the primary role of these scales is to measure the severity of depression and not to screen for and diagnose depression per se. This is a common misuse of both these scales in clinical practice. Even in the original article by Alexopoulas et al. (1988), the authors state "The Cornell scale is a quantitative measure of depression. Although, its total scores correlate with the presence of depressive syndromes classified by RDC, the Cornel scale is not designed for the use as a diagnostic instrument".

Another such scale, *Confusion Assessment Methodology* (CAM) is used to screen for delirium in hospitalized non-cognitively impaired older adults (Inouye et al., 1999). Adaptations of CAM scale have been validated (CAM-ICU) for non-verbal, ventilated patients in ICU settings. This and other adaptations of CAM are modified to include a cognitive and functional assessment or detailed descriptors of the target population and not the CAM criteria themselves (Inouye et al., 1999). However, these modifications unfortunately are only valid for non-premorbidly cognitively impaired older adults and in ICU setting only. CAM has also been suggested as a standardized screening tool for older adults with mild dementia/NCD (Morandi et al., 2012). Disorganized thinking, one of the key features of delirium, is very common in moderate to advanced stages of dementia/NCD. Even the most experienced clinician may find detecting changes in disorganized thinking, from baseline, to be extremely challenging. Reliability and validity of CAM in moderate to advanced stages of dementia/NCD is yet to be determined. Hence even with this scale the clinician is no further ahead in regards to attempts to rule in or out the clinical condition of delirium from BPSD.

Further yet, the *Neuropsychiatric Inventory* and the *Behavioral Pathology in Alzheimer Disease Rating Scale* have both been used to detect psychotic and other disruptive symptoms in individuals with dementia/NCD (de Medeiros, 2010). However, during advanced stages of dementia/NCD, when clinical examination becomes unreliable and the incidence for non-cognitive symptoms increases, the reliability of these scales in distinguishing a clinical state from a clinical condition is unknown (de Medeiros, 2010).

Current Models of Behaviors in Dementia/NCD

The literature is dichotomous along the biological versus psychosocial continuum models for the presence of behaviors in patients with dementia/NCD. The biological perspective to describe behaviors in dementia/NCD consists of the *continuum of agitation into aggression* model and the psychosocial perspective consists of *needs based Dementia compromised behaviors* model.

Continuum of Agitation into Aggression

This biologically-based model theorizes that aggression is the result of escalated agitation (Bédard et al., 1997). Based upon Cohen-Mansfield's research, the literature defines aggression as a component of agitation (Buhr & White, 2006). Bédard et al. (1997) proposed patients with dementia/NCD rarely display sporadic episodes of aggression and these episodes often occur due to the escalation of an agitated behavior. Several factors are known to exacerbate a state of agitation into a state of aggression. These are inclusive of physiological factors, such as appetite, thirst, fatigue, and need for mental and social stimulation, and health status, inclusive of medical and mental health (Kovach et al., 2005).

An additional way to conceptualize the cyclic nature of the continuum of agitation to aggression is on the basis of dementia/NCD patients' loss of insight and loss of self-awareness and monitoring regarding the regulation of their emotions and actions (Word Health Organization, 2012). Thereby, a patient with dementia/NCD may be unaware of the extent of loss of emotional control and, as a consequence, the degree of agitation leading to the emergence of aggressive behaviors.

Yet another hypothesis of a cycle of continuum of agitation to aggressive behavior was put forth by Fabiano (1996). According to this hypothesis, a "circumstantial episode" refers to any situation that further confuses a cognitively impaired individual. The confusion leads to a sense of loss of control, which may push the individual's state of anxiety to a state of panic (Fabiano, 1996). The sense of loss of control can pertain to one's own actions or thoughts, the actions of others, or the environment itself. The outcome is the occurrence of "aggressive behaviors, wandering behavior or a withdrawn response" (Fabiano, 1996). Any of these behaviors can become a part of a new circumstantial episode and give rise to the development of secondary behaviors.

Needs Driven Dementia Compromised Behaviors

The first of the psychosocial models for understanding behaviors in dementia/NCD was put forth by Algase et al. (1996), referred to as "unmet needs-based" behaviors. This model was later modified by Kovach et al. (2005) and titled "needs based dementia comprised" behaviors (C-NDB). This model theorizes that "background factors" and "proximal factors" interact to generate unmet needs (Kovach et al., 2005). Such an unmet need leads to generation of behaviors to satiate the needs. If this happens the behavior will stabilize. However, if the underlying needs are not met, primary behaviors will interact with personal, care, and contextual factors to generate secondary needs based behaviors.

Limitations of Current Models of Behaviors

Apart from limitations in current terminology, further complexities arise from the fact that all understanding of occurrence of behaviors is dichotomized along biological and psychosocial paradigms. Major strides have been made in the treatment of psychiatric illnesses, with restoration of function, only with a biopsychosocial (BPS) approach to understanding of these disorders (Dupuis et al., 2004). Why should we think any differently in managing behaviors in dementia/NCD? The literature consistently identifies a complex interplay amongst biological, personal (psychological) and environmental (social) factors for the generation of behaviors in dementia/NCD (Royall, 1994). Furthermore, in the absence of a BPS model for occurrence of behaviors in dementia/NCD, a comprehensive classification system cannot be developed, especially when it comes to understanding the meaning of behaviors in moderate to advanced dementia/NCD. A comprehensive model which incorporates biological, personal and environmental factors in the generation of behaviors in dementia/NCD is yet to be developed.

Conclusion

As long as a patient is able to participate in a reliable and valid clinical interview, it is possible to tease out individual syndromal presentations in accordance with established DSM-5 criteria. With the progression of dementia/NCD to moderate and advanced stages and when a valid and a reliable clinical assessment cannot be conducted, it becomes challenging to achieve the aforementioned. Review of the literature shows that, to date, under these circumstances, terminology has been used interchangeably and without precision. Literature has repeatedly demonstrated a relative paucity of reliable and valid assessment scales to clarify phenomenology, accurately diagnose and distinguish amongst clinical states or clinical conditions in patients with moderate to advanced stages of dementia/NCD (Morandi et al., 2012). This makes the accuracy of the diagnosis of BPSD, as it is one of exclusion, questionable in any patient with moderate to advanced dementia/NCD. Attempts to cluster individual behavioral symptoms into identifiable syndromes, using aforementioned standardized scales, either on the basis of a consistent temporal course or response to a common treatment intervention, for moderate to advanced dementia/NCD have failed the test of scientific rigor (Robert et al., 2010). As a result, it significantly limits our ability to extrapolate any meaningful conclusions from such studies.

The absence of a BPS model for occurrence of behaviors as a "common reference point" has further limited the development of a reliable and valid classification system for behaviors in patients with moderate to advanced dementia/NCD. As a result, it has prevented the development of a systematic methodology to identify such modifiable syndromes in moderate to advanced stages of dementia/NCD. This has been the primary reason for lack of significant progress in the development of new pharmacological and non-pharmacological treatment interventions for management of behaviors in moderate to advanced dementia/NCD. Identification of such modifiable syndromes in varied medical illnesses, regardless of etiology, has been the primary reasons for innovation of novel pharmacological and non-pharmacological intervention. It is such an approach which has resulted in progress made in management of all types of medical illnesses with restoration of function.

As a way forward, current literature on behaviors is urging clinicians to find the "meaning" for behaviors to be better managed, especially in moderate to advanced dementia/NCD (Kovach et al., 2005). It is proposed that a better understanding of meaning of behaviors should lead to consistent identification and labeling of individual behavioral symptoms. Such a consistent understanding of behaviors in moderate to advanced dementia/NCD should allow for a uniform aggregation of individual behavioral symptoms such that they can be evaluated for their consistency along temporal lines or response to a common therapeutic agent. This may facilitate the development and evaluation of novel pharmacological and non-pharmacological treatments in patients with moderate to advanced dementia/NCD.

The literature acknowledges these deficiencies in the existing terminology and classifications and does provide a way forward. Davis et al. (1997) published an innovative paper to address the reasons for heterogeneity in use of terminology and classification of behaviors in patients with dementia/NCDs. Davis et al. (1997) proposed that, "there is no single, universally accepted measure or methodology for operationalizing responsive behaviors, and variations in definition and measurement across studies have limited investigators' ability to draw meaningful conclusions about these behaviors". Davis et al. (1997) have identified five variables which contribute to the above-stated challenge:

- Shifting domain of problem behaviors
- Slippage across research constructs
- Unexplored rater bias
- Scoring bias
- Absence of benchmarking studies

Almost a decade later, Buhr and White (2006) reiterated the persistence of the same ambiguity in interpretation of present terminology, interchangeable use of terms and varied interpretations.

Reference Terminology

Acknowledging these deficits, adhering to the academic definitions of *Reference Terminology and Classification Systems* as well as constructs put forth by Davis et al. (1997) the following approach is being proposed as a way to forward.

Reference terminology is defined as "a set of concepts and relationships that provide a common reference point for comparisons and aggregation of data" (Imel & Campbell, 2003). When this definition is applied to the development of a comprehensive biopsychosocial (BPS) model for the occurrence of behaviors in dementia/NCD, one has to take into consideration the complex interplay amongst biological, psychological (personal) and social (environmental) factors identified to be contributory to generation of behaviors in dementia/NCD.

This model and terminology is based on the premise that behaviors in dementia/NCDs are influenced by the following:

Biological Factors

i. Stage of the disease (correlations with the changes in brain morphology and neurotransmitter functioning)
ii. Inherent Circadian Rhythms (CR)
iii. Innate Physiological Needs (PN)

Personal Factors

i. Pre-morbid personality which determine psychological defense mechanisms
ii. Acquired coping strategies

Environmental Factors

i. Milieu Structure (MS)
ii. Interpersonal Interactions (IPI)

This new BPS model for occurrence of behaviors is being labeled "Stage Congruent Response Behaviors" (SCRB - pronounced "scrub"). Chapter 3 elaborates on each of the above aforementioned variables and identifies the dynamic interaction amongst all of them. This dynamic interaction is being used to generate a comprehensive BPS model for occurrence of behaviors in patients with dementia/NCD.

Classification Systems

A *classification system* is defined as *"a systematic arrangement into classes or groups based on perceived common characteristics; a means of giving order to a group of disconnected facts. The groups or classes may have similar or like characteristics or may even be synonymous"* (Imel & Campbell, 2003). Davis et al. (1997) proposed a set of criteria, based upon these definitions, and as a way of developing a more reliable and valid measure of classification of behaviors in dementia/NCDs. These criteria are as follows:

    i.   Identification of target population
    ii.   Construction of items into categories which adequately represent the domain
   iii.   Definition of the purpose of the measure
   iv.   Specification of the construct of the category or domain

Identification of Target Population

The target population includes dementia/NCD patients with moderate to advanced stages of the disease. These patients are unable to participate in a valid and reliable clinical interview.

Construction of Items into Categories

This step involves recognition of individual behavioral symptoms and clustering them into clinically meaningful categories. Each clinical category is titled to adequately represent the symptoms collected therein.

Definition of the Purpose of the Measure

Defining the meaning and specific purpose of the behavior and how it serves the patient. Each clinical category identified will represent a specific purpose being served for the patient exhibiting the constellation of individual behavioral symptoms represented therein. Recent literature on behaviors is urging clinicians to find a meaning for behaviors in order to better understand behaviors (Kovach et al., 2005). It is proposed a better understanding of behaviors should lead to more optimal treatment interventions.

Specification of the Construct of Each Category

This criterion refers to putting forth of the theoretical constructs upon which the existence of each clinical behavioral category can be justified. These theoretical constructs are to be derived from existing literature. The dementia/NCD, behavioral, and developmental psychology literature provides abundant information on these theoretical constructs. These constructs are to help with the justification of the grouping of individual symptoms under each clinically meaningful category and the creation of individual behavioral category.

The criteria and format was chosen due to its relevance in classifying behavioral symptoms in dementia/NCD and its widespread acceptability. It is commonly cited and used in research regarding behaviors in persons with dementia/NCD or related mental health disorders. Its application to behavioral management of dementia/NCD and related mental health disorders in acute and long term care settings is ideal.

In practice, such an exercise should start by collection of a database of all observed signs and symptoms of behaviors in patients with moderate to advanced stage of dementia/NCD. Once a large enough database has been collected, similar or alike symptoms will be manually stratified into clusters. Each of these clusters should be able to represent a "clinically meaningful" category of behaviors in patients with dementia/NCD. Furthermore, each of these clinical categories should be justifiable on the basis of theoretical constructs derived from existing literature.

The author has been involved in this exercise for the last 5 years and proposes a new method for classification of behaviors in patients with moderate to advanced stages of dementia/NCD. From existing literature, the following theoretical constructs have been identified as the "specification of the construct" for each behavioral category developed:

- Behaviors based in information processing theories
- Behaviors based in motivational and needs based theories
- Behaviors based in theories on regulation of emotions
- Behaviors based in theories on principles of compliance and aggression
- Heterogeneous group which encompasses behavioral categories requiring a combination of the above theories

Behavioral categories represented under each of the above constructs are:

1. Behaviors based in Information Processing Theory (Chapter 4)
   a) Disorganized Behaviors
   b) Misidentification Behaviors
2. Behaviors based in Needs based and Motivational Theories (Chapter 5)
   a) Apathy Behaviors
   b) Goal Directed Behaviors
   c) Motor Behaviors
   d) Importuning Behaviors
3. Behaviors based in Theories on Regulation of Emotions (Chapter 6)
   a) Emotional Behaviors

    b)   Fretful/Trepidated Behaviors
4. Behaviors based in Theories on Principles of Compliance (Chapter 7)
    a)   Oppositional Behaviors
    b)   Physically Aggressive Behaviors
5. Behaviors based in Heterogeneous Group (Chapter 8)
        a)   Vocal Behaviors
        b)   Sexual Behaviors

References

Alexopoulos, G. S., Abrams, R. C., Young, R. C., & Shamoian, C. A. (1988).
    Cornell scale for depression in dementia. *Biological psychiatry*, 23, 271-
    284.
    doi: 10.1016/0006-3223(88)90038-8.
Algase, D.L., Beck, C., Kolanowski, A., Whall, A., Berent, S., Richards, K. &
    Beattie, E. (1996). Need-driven dementia-compromised behavior: An
    alternative view of disruptive behavior. *American Journal of Alzheimer's
    Disease   and   Other   Dementias*,   11,   10-19.   doi:
    10.1177/153331759601100603.
Alzheimer Knowledge Exchange Resource Centre. (2013) *About - Behavioural
    Supports Ontario*. Available from:
    http://www.akeresourcecentre.org/BSOAbout
Alzheimer Society. (2005) *POSITION PAPER ON THE CASA VERDE JURY
    RECOMMENDATIONS*. Available from:
    http://www.alzheimer.ca/on/~/media/Files/on/PPPI%20Documents/Posit
    ion-Paper-Casa-Verde-Jury-Sept05.ashx
American Psychiatric Association. (2000). *Diagnostic and statistical manual of
    mental disorders*, 4th edition. Washington, DC: Author.
American Psychiatric Association (Ed.). (2000). *Diagnostic criteria from DSM-
    IV-TR*. Amer Psychiatric Pub Incorporated.
Ballard, C., Gray, A. & Ayre, G. (1999). Psychotic symptoms, aggression and
    restlessness in dementia. *Revue neurologique*, 155, 4S44-4S52.
Bédard, M., Molloy, D.W., Pedlar, D., Lever, J.A. & Stones, M.J. (1997). 1997
    IPA/Bayer Research Awards in Psychogeriatrics - (secondplace).
    Associations between dysfunctional behaviors, gender, and burden in
    spousal caregivers of cognitively impaired older adults. *International
    Psychogeriatrics*, 9, 277-290. doi: 10.1017/S1041610297004444.
Black, W. & Almeida, O.P. (2004). A systematic review of the association
    between the behavioral and psychological symptoms of dementia and
    burden of care. *International Psychogeriatrics*, 16, 295-315. doi:
    10.1017/S1041610204000468.
Buhr, G. T., & White, H. K. (2006). Difficult behaviors in long-term care patients
    with dementia. *Journal of the American Medical Directors
    Association*, 7, 180-192. doi: 10.1016/j.jamda.2005.12.003.
Chenoweth, L., King, M. T., Jeon, Y. H., Brodaty, H., Stein-Parbury, J., Norman,
    R., Haas, M., & Luscombe, G. (2009). Caring for Aged Dementia Care
    Resident Study (CADRES) of person-centred care, dementia-care

mapping, and usual care in dementia: a cluster-randomised trial. *The Lancet Neurology*, 8, 317-325. doi: 10.1016/S1474-4422(09)70045-6.

Cohen-Mansfield, J. & Billig, N. (1986). Agitated behaviors in the elderly. I. A conceptual review. *Journal of the American Geriatrics Society*, 34, 711-721.

Cohen-Mansfield, J. (2003) Consent and Refusal in Dementia/NCD research: Conceptual and practical considerations. *Alzheimer's Disease and Associated*Disorders, 17, 17 - 25.

Corbett, A., Smith, J., Creese, B., & Ballard, C. (2012). Treatment of behavioral and psychological symptoms of Alzheimer's disease. *Current treatment options in neurology*, 14, 113-125. doi: 10.1007/s11940-012-0166-9.

Davis, L.L., Buckwalter, K. & Burgio, L.D. (1997). Measuring problem behaviors in dementia: Developing a methodological agenda. *Advances in Nursing Science*, 20, 40-55.

de Medeiros, et al. (2010). The Neuropsychiatric Inventory-Clinician rating scale (NPI-C): reliability and validity of a revised assessment of neuropsychiatric symptoms in dementia. *International Psychogeriatrics*, 22, 984-999.

Dupuis, S.L., Wiersma, E., & Loiselle, L. (2004). *The nature of responsive behaviors in long-term care settings*. Waterloo, ON: Murray Alzhiemer Research and Education Program.

Fabiano, L. (1996). Preventing Alzheimer's aggression: Supportive therapy in action. Edgewater, Fla: FCS Publications.

Finkel, & Burns. (1999) Consensus Group Definition. *International Psychogeriatric Association.* 5

Folstein, M. F., Folstein, S. E., & McHugh, P. R. (1975). "Mini-mental state": a practical method for grading the cognitive state of patients for the clinician. *Journal of psychiatric research*, *12*(3), 189-198.

Hamilton, P., Harris, D., & Le Clair, K. (2006). Putting the PIECES together: Learning program for professionals providing long-term care to older adults with cognitive/mental health needs.

Human Resources and Skills Development Canada. (2013). *Indicators of Well-being in Canada, Canadians in Context – Aging Population.* Available from: http://www4.hrsdc.gc.ca/.3ndic.1t.4r@-eng.jsp?iid=33

Imel, M. & Campbell, J.R. (2003). *Mapping from a Clinical Terminology to a Classification*. Available from: http://library.ahima.org/xpedio/groups/public/documents/ahima/bok1_02 2744.hcsp?dDocName=bok1_022744

Inouye, S.K., Schlesinger, M.J. & Lydon, T.J. (1999). Delirium: A symptom of how hospital care is failing older persons and a window to improve quality of hospital care, *American Journal of Medicine*, 106, 565-573. *Alzheimer's research & therapy*, 2, 24. doi:10.1186/alzrt48.

Kaplan, H. I., & Sadock, B. J. (1995). Comprehensive textbook of psychiatry, 6th ed. Baltimore: Williams and Wilkins.

Kovach, C.R., Noonan, P.E., Schlidt, A.M. & Wells, T. (2005). A model of consequences of need-driven, dementia-compromised behavior. *Journal of Nursing Scholarship*, 37, 134-140.

Liperoti, R., Pedone, C., & Corsonello, A. (2008). Antipsychotics for the treatment of behavioral and psychological symptoms of dementia (BPSD). *Current neuropharmacology*, *6*, 117. doi: 10.2174/157015908784533860.

Livingston, G., Johnston, K., Katona, C., Paton, J., & Lyketsos, C. G. (2005). Systematic review of psychological approaches to the management ofneuropsychiatric symptoms of dementia. *American Journal of Psychiatry*, 162, 1996-2021.

Madhusoodanan, S., Shah, P., Brenner, R., & Gupta, S. (2007). Pharmacological treatment of the psychosis of Alzheimer's Disease. *CNS drugs*, *21*(2), 101-115.

McShane, R. (2000). What Are the Syndromes of Behavioral and Psychological Symptoms of Dementia?. *International Psychogeriatrics*, *12*(S1), 147-153.

Morandi, A., McCurley, J., Vasilevskis, E.E., Fick, D.M., Bellelli, G., Lee, P., Jackson, J.C., Shenkin, S.D., Marcotrabucchi, Schnelle, J., Inouye, S.K., Ely, W.E. & MacLullich, A. (2012). Tools to detect delirium superimposed on dementia: A systematic review. *Journal of the American Geriatrics Society*, 60, 2005-2013.doi: 10.1111/j.1532-5415.2012.04199.x.

Ontario Ministry of Health and Long-term Care. (2005). *Handbook of Limited Use Drug Products*. Available from: http://www.health.gov.on.ca/en/pro/programs/drugs/formulary/limited_u se/limited_use_092705.pdf

Patel, V. & Hope, R.A. (1992) A rating scale for aggressive behaviour in the elderly - the RAGE. *Psychological medicine*, 22, 211-221.

Pulsford, D., & Duxbury, J. (2006). Aggressive behaviour by people with dementia in residential care settings: a review. *Journal of psychiatric and mental health nursing*, 13, 611-618.

Robert, P., Ferris, S., Gauthier, S., Ihl, R., Winblad, B., & Tennigkeit, F. (2010). Review of Alzheimer's disease scales: is there a need for a new multi-domain scale for therapy evaluation in medical practice?. *Alzheimer's research & therapy*, 2, 24. doi:10.1186/alzrt48.

Royall, D. R. (1994). Precis of executive dyscontrol as a cause of problemb in dementia. *Experimental aging research*, 20, 73-94.

Schnaider Beeri, M., Werner, P., Davidson, M., & Noy, S. (2002). The cost of behavioral and psychological symptoms of dementia (BPSD) in community dwelling Alzheimer's disease patients. *International journal of geriatric psychiatry*, 17, 403-408.

Scottish Intercollegiate Guidelines Network. (2006) *Management of Patients with Dementia*. Available from: http://www.sign.ac.uk/pdf/sign86.pdf

Seitz, D. P., Gill, S. S., Herrmann, N., Brisbin, S., Rapoport, M. J., Rines, J., Wilson, K., Le Clair, K., & Conn, D.K. (2013). Pharmacological treatments for neuropsychiatric symptoms of dementia in long-term care: A systematic review. *International Psychogeriatrics,* 25, 185-203. doi:10.1017/S1041610212001627.

Smith, M. & Buckwalter, K. (2005). Behaviors associated with dementia. *American Journal of Nursing*, 105, 40-52.

Speziale, J., Black, E., Coatsworth-Puspoky, R., Ross, T., & O'Regan, T. (2009). Moving forward: Evaluating a curriculum for managing responsive behaviors in a geriatric psychiatry inpatient population. *The Gerontologist*, *49*(4), 570-576.

Teri, L., Gibbons, L. E., McCurry, S. M., Logsdon, R. G., Buchner, D. M., Barlow, W. E., Kukull, W.A., LaCroix, A.Z., McCormick, & W., Larson, E.B. (2003). Exercise plus behavioral management in patients with Alzheimer disease: a randomized controlled trial. *JAMA: the journal of the American Medical Association*, 290, 2015-22.

Tolkien, J. R. R. (1954). The Fellowship of the Ring (Norwalk, Conn.)

Wetterling, T., Kanitz, R. D., & Borgis, K. J. (1994). The ICD-10 criteria for vascular dementia. *Dementia/NCD and Geriatric Cognitive Disorders*, *5*(3-4), 185-188.

World Health Organization. (2012). *World Alzheimer Report 2012, A public health priority*. Available from: http://whqlibdoc.who.int/publications/2012/9789241564458_eng.pdf

Chapter 3: Stage Congruent Responsive Behaviors (SCRB): A New Terminology to Label Behaviors in Dementia/NCD

Introduction

Current published models for understanding the presence of behaviors in patients with dementia/NCD, however, seem to be dichotomous along the biological versus psychosocial continuum. The biological model is represented by the *Continuum of Agitation into Aggression* model (Bédard et al., 1997) and the psychosocial model consists of *Needs Based Dementia Compromised Behaviors* (Kovach et al., 2005). Despite the fact literature identifies a tertiary approach inclusive of biological, personal (or psychological), and environmental (or social) factors as being contributory to the generation of behaviors in patients with dementia/NCD (Royall, 1994); neither of these existing models has incorporated aforementioned identified biological, personal (psychological) and environmental (social) factors in their formulation.

Factors Influencing Behaviors in Dementia/NCDs

The generation of behaviors in dementia/NCDs are influenced by the following biological, personal (psychological), and environmental (social) factors and are specific to the stage of the illness.

I.   Biological Factors
      a.   Stage of the disease (SOD)
      b.   Inherent Circadian Rhythms (CR)
      c.   Innate Physiological Needs (PN)
II.   Personal Factors
      a.   Pre-morbid personality which determine psychological defence mechanisms
      b.   Acquired coping strategies
III. Environmental Factors
      a.   Milieu Structure (MS)
      b.   Interpersonal Interactions (IPI)

The Role of Biological Factors

Biological factors which influence dementia/NCD include the stage of the disease, inherent circadian rhythms, and innate physiological needs.

Stage of the Disease (SOD)

Behavioral symptom profile in patients with Dementia/NCD of the Alzheimer's type (DAT) and Vascular Dementia/NCD (VaD) show significant overlap and occur later in the disease (Frédéric & Cummings, 2002). Changes in personality and behaviors in patients with frontal lobe dementia/NCD are distinct from those occurring in DAT and VaD and emerge in the early stages of the disease; often prior to the onset of cognitive impairment (Frédéric & Cummings, 2002). Severity of dementia/NCD, as measured by cognitive deficits, has been correlated with the presence of neuro-pathological findings in the brain (Frédéric & Cummings, 2002). Nevertheless, there are no correlations between "specific behavioral sets" and anatomical impairment in specific regions of the brain (Rosen et al. 2002). There is, however, a co-relationship between anatomical pathology and incidence of behaviors in patients with dementia/NCD (Förstl et al., 1993). Förstl et al. (1993) developed a PAC-score (summation score of physical disability (P), apathy (A) and communication failure (C)) which co-related lower brain weight, higher cortical tangle density, and greater neuronal loss in the hippocampus and nucleus basalis of Meynert with a higher incidence of BPSD.

Type of mood symptoms has also been noted to change with progression in the stages of dementia/NCD (Forsell et al., 1993; Rosenberg & Lyketsos, 2008). The presence of mood symptoms as a prodrome to developing Alzheimer's dementia/NCD has been established in several studies (Price & Morris 1999; Rosenberg & Lyketsos, 2008). Price & Morris (1999) have demonstrated that some of the first neuro-pathological changes in the brain are present for up to 10 years before a diagnosis of dementia/NCD is made; which may correlate with prodromal depressive symptoms. There is a higher prevalence of dysthymic disorder in patients with mild dementia/NCD in comparison to age matched controls (Payne et al. 2002). Payne et al. (2002) also reported that depression afflicted a considerable proportion of long-term care residents with dementia/NCD; often with moderate to advanced stages. Additionally, according to Forsell et al. (1993), "dysphoria, appetite disturbance, feelings of guilt, and thoughts of death/suicidal ideation" are prevalent in mild to moderate stages of the disease. Motivational disturbances of decreased energy, interest levels, concentration, and thinking occur in the moderate to advanced stages of dementia/NCD (Forsell et al., 1993). These studies support the notion that the type of depressive symptoms changes with the progression of dementia/NCD.

Symptoms of anxiety are often viewed as an adaptation to the stress of being diagnosed with dementia/NCD at the beginning of the disease. Such patients are aware of their deficits and respond accordingly with fear over a future filled with uncertainty. Patients with dementia/NCD diagnosed with generalized anxiety disorder often do not show these symptoms before the onset of dementia/NCD; thereby suggesting a complex interplay of biopsychosocial variables (Porter et al., 2003). Anxiety symptoms also continue in the latter stages of the disease, when all measurable evidence of awareness of deficits and the ability to form any type of cognitive schema is lost.

Similar evidence exists regarding the prevalence of psychotic symptoms in the progression of dementia/NCD; there is an absence of psychotic symptoms in the early stages of dementia/NCD (World Health Organization, 2012). Delusional Misidentification Syndrome (DMS), delusions and hallucinations are often present in the moderate stage of Alzheimer's disease, with all such symptoms abating in the end stages (International Psychogeriatrics Association, 2002). This suggests a threshold degree of cognitive disturbance is required for psychotic symptoms to develop (Lyketsos et al., 2002). With the disease progression, a degree of cognitive preservation may be required for these symptoms to develop and a severely impaired brain, as in the advanced stage of dementia/NCD, is incapable of forming these symptoms.

The above speaks to the presence of neuropsychiatric symptoms as a prodrome to or sequlae of dementia/NCD in patients without psychiatric co-morbidity. There are, however, many patients with adult onset psychiatric illness who later go on to develop dementia/NCD. The role of co-morbid psychiatric illness as a risk factor for developing cognitive impairment is increasingly being recognized (Artero et al., 2008). In such patients, the quality of pre-existing psychiatric symptom presentation in the acute phase of their primary psychiatric illness may not be lost when these patients go on to develop dementia/NCD. In fact, the behavioral symptoms emerging in these patients will often be influenced and modified by the nature of the primary psychiatric illness. Collecting information, therefore, on the symptom presentation of the primary co-morbid psychiatric illness, in the acute phase of relapse, should help better identify and understand behaviors in these patients as they go on to develop dementia/NCD. To enhance practice, the clinical approach needs to encompass an understanding of the sign and symptoms of the underlying psychiatric disease and how it may be shaping and influencing presenting behaviors in dementia/NCD

In summary, the quality of mood, anxiety, and psychotic symptoms are influenced by the stages and progression of dementia/NCD. The presence of pre-existing psychiatric co-morbid illness is not only a risk factor to developing dementia/NCD, but also shapes behavioral symptom manifestation if these patients go on to develop dementia/NCD.

Inherent Circadian Rhythms (CR)

Bodily functions show variability over a 24 hour day in a cyclical manner. Examples of such predictable cyclical changes include heart rate, blood pressure, body temperature, bowel function, and level of arousal. This is referred to as Circadian Rhythm (CR). All of these cyclical changes have been correlated with changes in hormonal levels, such as cortisol, melatonin, TSH and testosterone; neurotransmitters, such as serotonin, dopamine, norepinephrine, and acetylcholine; and digestive enzymes (Van Cauter, 1990; Sensi, Palitti & Guagnano, 1993; Czeisler & Klerman, 1999). CR is influenced by external or exogenous variables in the *environment* yet remain independently governed by all the above endogenous variables. These exogenous variables include, but are not exclusive of; medications, nutritional and hormonal supplements, environmental manipulation of light, color, changes in shift times of the nurses, and additional variables described under the "Environmental Factors" section of this article. The same principles are applicable to patients in non-institutional settings.

CR also influences various cognitive and emotional measures in humans as these measures show change in a circadian manner. Motor performance, memory, cognitive speed, reaction times, and even mood show this predictable variability over a 24 hour day. As a consequence, inherent changes in CR are likely to have a direct and congruent impact on any variety of behaviors emerging in patients with dementia/NCD. In addition to within 24 hour day variability, there is day-to-day and week-to-week variability in CR and their congruent influence on behavioral symptoms emerging in dementia/NCD patients.

Consequently, two sets of observations are made in patients with dementia/NCD exhibiting behavioral symptoms:

1. Diurnal variation of symptoms during the course of the day
2. Inherent cycling of behaviors over days and weeks

Examples of the above two are seen in a wide variety of behavioral symptoms and inclusive of; disruptive vocalization, wandering, exit seeking, agitation, and sleep schedule disturbances. Such a diurnal variation is commonly referred to as "sun-downing".

Innate Physiological Needs (PN)

Important natural physiological changes occur in the body throughout the course of each day. Fatigue with the need to rest and sleep; pain, or discomfort and seeking relief (not necessarily through the use of medications), hunger, thirst and seeking satiation, the need to void and/or defecate, and the need for mental and social stimulation to stay connected with the environment are all factors which influence the way in which an individual conducts themselves during the day . If these innate PN remain unmet, they will influence any subsequent generation of behaviors. Variations and limitations in satiation of these innate PN, either individual or collectively on, within-in day, or day to day basis, will influence behaviors accordingly.

Relationship between CR and Innate PN

Disruptions in CR are inherent to the advancement of the disease of dementia/NCD. Such disruptions in CR will congruently impact on innate PN. Depending upon whether the PN has been fulfilled or not, will in turn, impact on the regulation of CR. Examples to support this dynamic interaction are reviewed below.

Disruption in CR can result in dysregulation of sleep schedule. This dysregulation can take the form of increased duration of wakefulness at night; overall decrease in sleep time; increased napping throughout the day; and an overall phase-disrupted sleep-wake schedule. This is likely to impact on the innate *PN* of the need to rest, erratic appetite and intake and the regulation of the need to void or defecate. Disruptions in these innate PN will further dys-regulate CR.

Another example of disruption in CR involves mental arousal. Diurnal variation in mental arousal will impact on cognitive and motor speed and its congruent impact on the need for mental stimulation. Decrease in arousal will result in a decrease in need for mental stimulation and an increase in arousal will result in an increased need for mental stimulation. Disruptions in the need for mental arousal will impact on the regulation of CR.

Conversely, changes in PN may impact on CR as well. In some patients, fecal loading may result in a decrease in mental arousal with congruent decrease in need for mental stimulation. In other patients, fecal impaction can result in increased mental arousal with congruent need for mental stimulation. Regulation of the bowels in both of these examples, by virtue of satiating the innate PN, will restore mental arousal. Inadequate bladder emptying, due to any etiology, will result in an increased post-void residual. This may result in increased discomfort and may even cause pain. This will result in an increase in mental arousal with a congruent increase in need of mental stimulation to satiate the need to fully empty the bladder. This may occur naturally due to retention with overflow or by therapeutic decompression. Once this occurs, the mental arousal returns to normal, and CR is restored. Hence, there is a dynamic relationship between CR and innate PN.

The Role of Personal Factors

Personal factors which influence dementia/NCD include pre-morbid personality, and acquired coping strategies.

Pre-morbid Personality

McCrae & John (1992) proposed a five (5) factor model of personality in healthy (non-cognitive impaired) individuals:

1. Neuroticism (emotional instability)
2. Extraversion (versus introversion)
3. Conscientiousness (rigidity vs. flexibility)
4. Agreeability (versus aggression)
5. Openness to experience

In times of stress, healthy individuals draw upon these innate personality factors to cope with any given situation. Depending upon which of the above individual personality factors are predominant in a given individual, cumulative coping responses over a life time may be adaptive or mal-adaptive. Unfortunately a preponderance of maladaptive coping mechanisms increases the vulnerability to emotional disorders in healthy individuals. Conversely, effective coping mechanisms assist in the protection against psychological problems (Riskind & Alloy, 2006). Hence, these personality traits or factors determine individual psychological defence mechanisms and acquired coping strategies exhibited by individuals in varied, stressful and non-stressful, social settings, including when the individual goes on to develop dementia/NCD.

Several studies have utilized this model to demonstrate a relationship between individual personality factor, aging with onset of cognitive impairment, and the prevalence of co-morbid psychiatric disorders. Agronin (1998) has discussed the important role of these personality factors in normal aging and cognitive decline associated with aging. Furukawa et al. (1998) has established a relationship between increased vulnerability to psychiatric illness with aging and individual pre-morbid personality traits. Amongst the traits researched, neuroticism, or emotional instability, is the most highly correlated with anxiety and depressive disorders in patients with dementia/NCD (Von Gunten, Pocnet & Rossier, 2009). Von Gunten, Pocnet and Rossier (2009) also found that patients who were more neurotic in their pre-morbid personality were usually more emotionally labile and tense when (later) suffering from dementia/NCD, showing a connection between pre-morbid personality traits and BPSD. Chaterjee et al. (1992) have shown an association between high levels of neuroticism and development of depression and high level of pre-morbid hostility with the development of delusions in patients with Alzheimer's dementia/NCD. Meins, Frey and Thiesemann (1998) have shown an association between high levels of neuroticism and conscientiousness (rigidity vs. flexibility) in pre-morbid personalities and development of behavioral symptoms in dementia/NCD.

As is evident from the preceding, pre-morbid personality traits increase the vulnerability to certain types of emotional disorders and this vulnerability is further heightened with the onset of cognitive impairment and its progression to dementia/NCD. This clearly demonstrates a dynamic relationship of personal factors with the progression of cognitive impairment for the entire duration of decline of the disease.

Acquired Coping Strategies

There is no universally accepted classification for coping mechanisms, though Weiten et al. (2009), has placed the most practical approach to understanding coping mechanisms. Weiten et al. (2009) identified three broad types of coping mechanisms: appraisal or adaptive cognitive focused, emotional focused, and problem focused. The first coping mechanism, "appraisal" or "adaptive cognitive focused" refers to individuals modifying the way they think about the problem on hand as a means of coping with it. Examples include using denial, minimizing or rationalizing a given situation. "Emotional focused", the second coping mechanism, refers to individuals using principles of emotional regulation as a means of coping with stress. Examples include managing hostile emotions, meditating or systemic relaxation techniques. The third and final coping mechanism "problem focused" refers to individuals using solution focused strategies as a means to cope. Individuals utilize these coping mechanisms, individually or in combination, to deal with the initial shock of diagnosis of dementia/NCD and subsequent progression of the disease.

It has been proposed the same neuro-pathological mechanisms responsible for cognitive decline also result in interruptions of the neuronal circuits involved in the regulation of the previously stated personality factors (Alves et al. 2009).

With onset and progression of cognitive impairment through various stages of dementia/NCD, there will be congruent changes in the identified personality factors. This, in turn, will impact on psychological defence mechanism and subsequently, the acquired coping strategies in patients with a progressive dementia/NCD. These changes are likely to influence and increase the vulnerability of patients to develop emotional and behavioral symptoms with the advancement of dementia/NCD.

In summary, pre-morbid personality traits increase the vulnerability to certain types of emotional disorders and it is further heightened with the onset of cognitive impairment and its progression through dementia/NCD. The same applies to regulation of acquired coping mechanisms. There is a dynamic relationship amongst "personal factors" (personality traits with psychological defence mechanisms and coping strategies) and the progression of cognitive impairment for the entire duration of decline of dementia/NCD.

The Role of Environmental Factors

Environmental factors consist of two distinct elements: milieu structure (MS) and interpersonal interactions (IPI).

Milieu Structure (MS)

There are aspects of MS which are *static* in nature and those which are *dynamic.* *"Static"* refers to the structural layout of the environment, inclusive of the design of the environment (e.g., amount of space, whether continuous or interrupted), type of furniture, lighting fixtures, color of the walls, décor on the walls and the type of flooring on the unit. There are other aspects of MS which are *"dynamic"* throughout the day such as the turning lighting on and off, placement and movement of furniture, continuous open and closing of main and individual room doors, the degree of cleanliness or clutter throughout the milieu and the type of music and television programming at different times of the day. Whereas, the static factors remain constant, dynamic factors tend to change on a day to day basis or within. These factors are applicable to patients residing in their residential home, a care home or hospital setting.

Interpersonal Interactions (IPI)

IPI can be *random* or *structured.* *"Random"* IPI would differ in a personal residence home versus care homes and hospitals. In residential homes, random IPI can take the form of visits from family and friends, community agency support workers and caregiver's demeanor. In care homes and in hospital settings, IPI is inclusive of changing patient population, changes in behaviors of co-patients, staff personal changes at shift times and on different days, activities of the cleaning staff, kitchen staff and food cart activities at meal and snack times, family members visiting at different times during visiting hours and the degree of crowding of the space with visitors as examples. *"Structured"* IPI can be available at home in the form of private one-on-one companion at times of occurrence of highest frequency and severity of behaviors. Structured IPI, in a care home or a hospital setting, can refer to the activities organized by recreation staff. Most specialised dementia/NCD behavior units have scheduled activities at those times of the day during higher level of intensity of behaviors as a means to manage. These activities are focused around specific meal times or change of staff at shift times; usually in the evenings between 4 p.m. to 11 p.m. Both random and structured IPI are dynamic in nature.

Relationship between MS and IPI

There is a relationship that exists between MS and IPI affecting the severity of behaviors exhibited in individuals with dementia/NCD.

Movement of patients exhibiting behaviors, within or between facilities, occurs for various reasons. Any of these individual changes are made with a view to diminishing behaviors and associated risks.

Reasons for such moves include:

1. Changes within the existing environment failed to reduce behaviors
2. To decrease caregiver and care provider burden and stress
3. The new ward may be better adapted to the type of behaviors being exhibited
4. To better fit in with other patients
5. Transfer to a hospital treatment setting to receive higher level of care

Any or all of the above changes will result in changing of MS (static and dynamic) and IPI (random and structured). These examples represent an absolute change in all of the environmental variables. The complex interplay amongst these variables influences behaviors, for better or worse. The above moves are made with the view of diminishing behaviors and associated risks. There could be varying degrees of change in external factors, such as only the dynamic aspect of MS changing; only random aspect of IPI changing; only the structured aspects of IPI changing; or any degree of permutation and combination of the variable on this continuum.

Biopsychosocial Responsive Model

There is a complex interaction amongst Biological, Personal and Environmental factors for the generation of behaviors in dementia/NCD. A *"responsive model"* is proposed to understand the generation of behaviors in patients with dementia/NCD. This *"responsive model"* has three component stages:

i. Input
ii. Processing
iii. Output

Input Stage

Internal and *External* factors form the input arm of the *"responsive model"*. *Internal factors (IF)* consist of CR and PN. *External factors (EF)* include *static* and *dynamic* aspects of MS and *random* and *structured* aspects of IPI. Internal and external factors are dynamic on with-in same day, day-to-day and a week to week basis. *Internal* and *External* factors represent into the processing stage of the *"responsive model"*. The information from the changes in the internal and external factors will be continuously inputted in to the processing phase of the *"responsive module"*.

Processing Stage

Processing of the information inputted via the *"internal"* and *"external"* factors is determined by the stage of dementia/NCD. This refers to the pattern and severity of cognitive impairment in a patient at that point in their illness. The severity of cognitive impairment can be mild, moderate or advanced. The staging of the disease is also a dynamic process and progression is mostly an insidious process except in an acute intracranial vascular event, infective or traumatic etiology. The insidious disease process is generally staged by assessing the patient every 6 to 12 months. The rate of progression of the disease will have a congruent impact on the functionality and adaptability, or impairment thereof, of "personal" factors. Hence, for a given stage of the disease, congruent changes in personal factors will leave the patient to navigate or adapt to the changing needs and demands of the internal and external factors. Therefore, stage congruent response is secondary to disease stage congruent processing. This is not unlike a computer. Older computers do not possess enough RAM to process the newer software (input). Thus, the output is specific to the amount of memory or the ability of the computer to process the new program, and thus may not have equivalent output.

According to the ecological model of aging proposed by Lawton (1974), behaviors are viewed as a dynamic interaction between the competence of an individual and their ability to deal with various aspects and demands from the environment. As used in this context, "competence" refers to the sum total of functioning of the biological and the personal factors in a given individual. Also according to Lawton's (1974) model, a patient with low competence put in an averagely demanding environment can produce behaviors to the same extent as a patient with an average competence put in a highly demanding environment.

Impairment in memory, visuospatial, and/or executive functions in dementia/NCD can lower the competency of the individual to negotiate the changing demands in the environment or change of environment. Additionally, if a patient with pre-existing comorbid psychiatric illness such as mood, anxiety, or psychotic disorder goes on to develop superimposed cognitive impairment, the vulnerability from the underlying psychiatric co-morbid illness will be compounded by cognitive impairment, thereby further decreasing the competence. Decreased competence will express itself through emergence of maladaptive coping mechanisms in times of stress, such as those posed by changes in the internal and external factors. All of these factors will accumulatively increase the likelihood of emergence of emotional and behavioral symptoms.

Output Stage

As is evident from above, the output of behaviors is the net result of a complex dynamic interaction amongst IF, EF, SOD, with or without prior mental illness, and its congruent impact on PF. The type of behaviors generated will be determined by the competence of the patient. The competence of the patient will be determined by the severity of CI, mild, moderate of severely demented, congruent changes in personal factors with, or without, the presence of prior mental illness.

For example, in the mild stages of dementia/NCD and the absence of previous mental illness, with congruent change in personal factors, there may be no behaviors exhibited in their home environment. This is due to familiarity of the milieu and people within it. Hence, the changes in various components of IPI and MS, on within day or day to day, basis is not perceived by the individual's current SOD to be a stressful state. As this patient's CI progresses competence is compromised and even the familiarity of the home no longer serves as a comfort. The patient will struggle with the changing demands of the MS and IPI with its congruent impact on CR and innate PN. This results in the generation of SCRB. Behaviors, for example, may take the form of waking up at 2 AM and getting "ready to go to work" or in the form of wanting to go home and attempting to exit-seek. As is evident, depending on the stage of the disease, the reduced competence is responsible for handling the information flowing in (IF and EF), thereby, influencing the quality of the behaviors resulting in a stage congruent response.

If the same patient were to be referred to a specialized day program, as a way of coping with caregiver stress, this would pose a new set of challenges and demands for the patient. MS and IPI have changed but the stage of the disease and its impact on competence has not. Changes in MS and IPI and the conspicuous absence of primary caregiver (possibly the spouse) will be processed by the brain with the expression of a quality of stage congruent response behaviors specific to the stage of the disease and ability to process. In this scenario, the behaviors may take the form of the patient repeatedly asking for his/her spouse to pick them up, shadowing and clinging to staff and appearing fretful.

Behaviors in the same patient are likely to change with a move into a LTC facility. Once again, components of MS and IPI have changed but the stage of the disease and its decreased competence has not. Changes in MS and IPI will have congruent impact on CR and innate PN. All of this information will processed by the SOD with its reduced competence thereby generating different quality of stage congruent response behaviors. Behaviors may take the form of moving furniture, packing and unpacking clothes and wanting to go home.

Once the patient has adapted to this MS and IPI, with its congruent impact in CR and innate PN, any further behaviors will be influenced by these set of IF and EF. As an example, a patient required moving to a different room due to a water leak. The EF consisted of view of snow on the ground outside, their room with an attached bathroom and burst pipes resulting in water on the floor. The behaviors which emerged, as a consequence, consisted of the patient wanting to go to the bank to pay the water utility bill. The behaviors could have also taken the form of wanting to go home to turn up the heating so as to prevent the water pipes from freezing.

In all of the above examples, it is how the information is processed by the cognitively impaired brain which determines the type of behaviors that emerge. Hence, SOD is responsible for determining the *quality* of behaviors. It is the *quality of* SCRB which are changing in the scenarios described above.

Quality of behaviors refers to the individual characteristics or description of the type of behaviors being observed in a patient with dementia/NCD. The *quality of behaviors* generated is primarily determined by the SOD (severity of cognitive impairment, with or without mental illness and congruent changes in PF).

Abnormalities in CR and or PN in this patient, in any of the above scenarios, would further influence behaviors. As an example, additional changes in bowels and or sleep rhythms will impact on the mental arousal and congruent need for, or lack thereof, mental stimulation. Fecal loading and sleep disruption will increase lethargy and decrease mental arousal. This will impact on the patient's interactions with MS and IPI. On the days when bowels and or sleep are regulated, the level of arousal and the need for mental stimulation is at a level which allows for appropriate interaction with MS and IPI. On the days of fecal loading or sleep disruption, there will be a decrease in the need for mental stimulation. Consequently, the interaction of the patient with its MS and IPI will be minimal on such days.

Hence, on days when the bowels are moving regularly or their sleep is regulated, adequate mental arousal will result in the generation of behaviors due to an active interaction between EF and SOD. On the days of fecal loading or sleep dysregulation, mental lethargy will not result in generation behaviors due to an absence of an active interaction between EF and SOD. Hence, changes in IF and EF are responsible for determining the changes in *frequency* and *duration* of behaviors on within day, day to day and week to week basis. Likewise, the *severity* of each *quality* of behaviors generated is also determined by the IF and EF.

Lastly, the behaviors, in themselves, will result in changes in aspects of the environment (IPI and some components of MS) along with impact on their PN and CR. These changes are fed back into the processing module via the input arm to continue to influence the generated behaviors. Hence, there is a continuous feedback loop with dynamic interaction at all different levels of the "input", "processing" and "output" stage of this responsive model.

Therefore, the term which most accurately reflects these complex interactions is: *Stage Congruent Responsive Behaviors (SCRB)..* The following diagram represents the schematic of the above principles described to support the terminology "*Stage Congruent Responsive Behaviors*" in dementia/NCD.

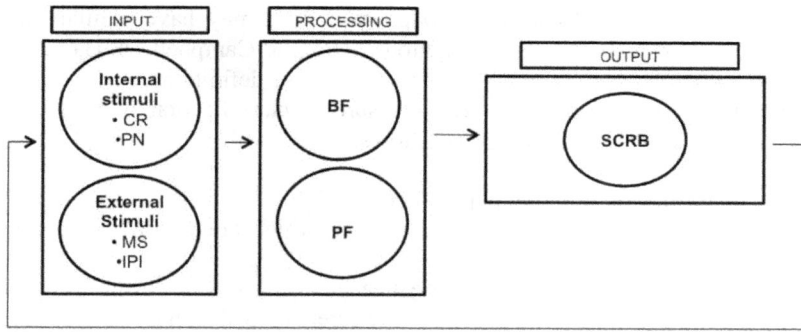

Figure 1 – Diagram of Stage Congruent Response Behaviors (SCRB) (Luthra 2012)

Figure 1 describes how biological, personal, and environmental factors of a person with dementia/NCD dynamically interact to result in a behavior. An internal (CR or PN) or external (MS or IPI) are inputted either separately or together, resulting in impaired processing through biological factors (e.g., the stage of the disease) and personal factors (e.g., coping mechanisms), resulting in an output of SCRB

Conclusion

Biological Factors (stage of the disease, presence or absence of mental illness, inherent circadian rhythms, and innate physiological needs), *Personal Factors* (Pre-morbid personality and acquired coping mechanisms) and *Environmental Factors* (milieu structure and Interpersonal Interactions) were all identified as playing a significant role in the generation of behaviors in patients with dementia/NCD. There is a complex interplay among these three factors in the generation of behaviors.

Stage of the disease refers to the severity of cognitive impairment. The stage of the disease (moderate or severe cognitive impairment) with congruent changes in personal factors, with a given set of internal and external factors, will generate a certain *quality* of behaviors. For the same patient, progression in the severity of cognitive impairment with congruent changes in personal factors, with a given set of internal and external factors, will change the *quality* of the behaviors. Hence, the *quality* of behaviors generated is a stage congruent phenomenon.

The *frequency*, *duration*, and *severity* of a given quality of behaviors will be influenced by the inherent fluctuations in CR and PN, which are, in turn, influenced by the changes in MS and IPI within environment in which the patient resides. Hence, the behaviors are a product of an interaction amongst all of these variables and responsive to changes in any/all of the variables. For these reasons, *Stage Congruent Responsive Behaviors (SCRB)* is the most appropriate terminology to label behaviors in patients with dementia/NCD.

Proposed Classification System for SCRB

A *classification system* is defined as "a systematic arrangement into classes or groups based on perceived common characteristics; a means of giving order to a group of disconnected facts. The groups or classes may have similar or like characteristics or may even be synonymous " (Imel & Campbell, 2003). Davis et al. (1997) proposed a set of criteria, based upon these definitions, and as a way of developing a more reliable and valid measure of classification of behaviors in dementia/NCDs. These criteria are as follows:

i.   Identification of target population
ii.   Construction of items into categories which adequately represent the domain
iii.   Definition of the purpose of the measure
iv.   Specification of the construct of the category or domain

Identification of Target Population

The target population includes dementia/NCD patients with moderate to advanced stages of the disease. These patients are unable to participate in a valid and reliable clinical interview.

Construction of Items into Categories

This step involves recognition of individual behavioral symptoms and clustering them into clinically meaningful categories. Each clinical category is titled to adequately represent the symptoms collected therein.

Definition of the Purpose of the Measure

Defining the meaning and specific purpose of the behavior and how it serves the patient. Each clinical category identified will represent a specific purpose being served for the patient exhibiting the constellation of individual behavioral symptoms represented therein. Recent literature on behaviors is urging clinicians to find a "meaning" for behaviors in order to better understand behaviors (Kovach et al., 2005). It is proposed a better understanding of behaviors should lead to more optimal treatment interventions.

Specification of the Construct of Each Category

This criterion refers to putting forth of the theoretical constructs upon which the existence of each clinical behavioral category can be justified. These theoretical constructs are to be derived from existing literature. Existing dementia/NCD, behavioral, and developmental psychology literature provides abundant information on these theoretical constructs. These constructs are to help with the justification of the grouping of individual symptoms under each clinically meaningful category and the creation of individual behavioral category.

      These criteria and format was chosen due to its relevancy in classifying behavioral symptoms in dementia/NCD and its widespread acceptability. It is commonly cited and used in research regarding behaviors in persons with dementia/NCD or related mental health disorders. Its application to behavioral management of dementia/NCD and related mental health disorders in acute and long term care settings is ideal.

In practice, such an exercise should start by collection of a data base of all observed signs and symptoms of behaviors in patients with moderate to advanced stage of dementia/NCD. Once a large enough data base has been collected, similar or alike symptoms will be manually stratified into clusters. Each of these clusters should be able to represent a "clinically meaningful" category of behaviors in patients with dementia/NCD. Furthermore, each of these clinical categories should be justifiable on the basis of theoretical constructs derived from existing literature.

The author has been involved in this exercise for the last 5 years and is proposing a new method for classification of behaviors in patients with moderate to advanced stages of dementia/NCD. From existing literature, the following theoretical constructs have been identified as the "specification of the construct" for each behavioral category developed:

- Behaviors based in Information Processing Theories
- Behaviors based in Motivational and Needs based Theories
- Behaviors based in Theories on Regulation of Emotions
- Behaviors based in Theories on Principles of Compliance and Aggression
- Heterogeneous Group which encompasses behavioral categories requiring a combination of the above Theories

Behavioral categories represented under each of the above constructs are:

Behaviors based in Information Processing Theory (Chapter 4)
  a) Disorganized Behaviors
  b) Misidentification Behaviors
Behaviors based in Needs based and Motivational Theories
(Chapter 5)
  a) Apathy Behaviors
  b) Goal Directed Behaviors
  c) Motor Behaviors
  d) Importuning Behaviors
Behaviors based in Theories on Regulation of Emotions (Chapter 6)
  a) Emotional Behaviors
  b) Fretful/Trepidated Behaviors
Behaviors based in Theories on Principles of Compliance
(Chapter 7)
  a) Oppositional Behaviors
  b) Physically Aggressive Behaviors

Behaviors based in Heterogeneous Group (Chapter 8)
a) Vocal Behaviors
b) Sexual Behaviors

References

Alves, G.S., Alves, C.E.O., Lanna, M.E.O., Ericeira-Valente, L., Sudo, F.K., Moreira, D., Engelhardt, E. & Laks, J. (2009). Clinical characteristics in subcortical ischemic white matter disease. *Arquivos de Neuro-Psiquiatria*, 67, 173-178. doi: 10.1590/S0004-282X2009000200001.

Agronin, M. E. (1998). Personality and psychopathology in late life. *Geriatrics*, 53, 35 - 40.

Artero S., et al. (2008). Risk profiles for mild cognitive impairment and progression to dementia are gender specific. *Journal of Neurology, Neurosurgery & Psychiatry*, 79, 979-984. doi: 10.1136/jnnp.2007.136903.

Bédard, M., Molloy, D.W., Pedlar, D., Lever, J.A. & Stones, M.J. (1997). 1997 IPA/Bayer Research Awards in Psychogeriatrics - (secondplace). Associations between dysfunctional behaviors, gender, and burden in spousal caregivers of cognitively impaired older adults. *International Psychogeriatrics*, 9, 277-290. doi: 10.1017/S1041610297004444.

Chatterjee A., Strauss M.E., Smyth K.A., & Whitehouse P.J. (1992). Personality changes in Alzheimer's disease. *Archives of Neurology*, 49, 486–491. doi: 10.1001/archneur.1992.00530290070014.

Czeisler, C. A., & Klerman, E. B. (1999). Circadian and sleep-dependent regulation of hormone release in humans. *Recent Progress in Hormone Research*, 54, 97-132.

Förstl, H., Burns, A., Levy, R., Cairns, N., Luthert, P., & Lantos, P. (1993). Neuropathological correlates of behavioural disturbance in confirmed Alzheimer's disease. *The British Journal of Psychiatry*, 163, 364-368. doi: 10.1192/bjp.163.3.364.

Forsell, Y., Jorm, A. F., Fratiglioni, L., Grut, M., & Winbald, B. (1993). Application of DSM-III-R criteria for major depressive episode to elderly subjects with and without dementia. *The American Journal of Psychiatry*, 150, 1199-1202.

Frédéric, A., & Cummings, J. L. (2002). Neuropsychiatric symptoms in the dementias. *Current Opinion in Neurology*, 15, 445-450.

Furukawa, T., Hori, S., Yoshida, S. I., Tsuji, M., Nakanishi, M., & Hamanaka, T. (1998). Premorbid personality traits of patients with organic (ICD-10 F0), schizophrenic (F2), mood (F3), and neurotic (F4) disorders according to the five-factor model of personality. *Psychiatry research*, 78, 179-187. doi: 10.1016/S0165-1781(98)00014-6.

Imel, M., & Campbell, J.R. (2003). *Mapping from a Clinical Terminology to a Classifcation*. AHIMA's 75th Anniversary National Convention and Exhibit Proceedings. Retrieved from: http://library.ahima.org/xpedio/idcplg?IdcService=GET_HIGHLIGHT_INFO&Q ueryText=(mapping+from+a+clinical+terminology+to+a+classification) %3Cand%3E(xPublishSite%3Csubstring%3E%60BoK%60)&SortField

=xPubDate&SortOrder=Desc&dDocName=bok1_022744&HighlightTy
pe=HtmlHighlight&dWebExtension=hcsp

International Psychogeriatric Association. (2002). *Module Two*, in *Behavioral and Psychological Symptoms of Dementia (BPSD) Educational Pack*. International Psychogeriatric Association, (IPA): Skokie, IL, USA.

Kovach, C.R., Noonan, P.E., Schlidt, A.M. & Wells, T. (2005). A model of consequences of need-driven, dementia-compromised behavior. *Journal of Nursing Scholarship*, 37, 134-140. doi: 10.1111/j.1547-5069.2005.00025_1.x.

Lawton, M. P. (1974). Social ecology and the health of older people. *American Journal of Public Health*, 64, 257-20. doi: 10.2105/AJPH.64.3.257.

Lyketsos, C. G., Lopez, O., Jones, B., Fitzpatrick, A. L., Breitner, J., & DeKosky, S. (2002). Prevalence of neuropsychiatric symptoms in dementia and mild cognitive impairment. *JAMA: the journal of the American Medical Association*, 288, 1475-1483. doi: 10.1001/jama.288.12.1475.

McCrae, R. R., & John, O. P. (1992). An introduction to the five-factor model and its applications. *Journal of personality*, 60, 175-215. doi: 10.1111/j.1467-6494.1992.tb00970.x.

Meins, W., Frey, A., & Thiesemann, R. (1998). Premorbid personality traits in Alzheimer's disease: Do they predispose to noncognitive behavioral symptoms? *International Psychogeriatrics*, 10, 369-378. doi: 10.1017/S1041610298005468.

Payne, J.L., Sheppard, J.M.E., Steinberg, M., Warren, A., Baker, A., Steele, C., Brandt, J. & Lyketsos, C.G. (2002). Incidence, prevalence and outcomes of depression in residents of a long-term care facility with dementia. *International Journal of Geriatric Psychiatry*, 17, 247-253. doi: 10.1002/gps.589.

Porter, V. R., Buxton, W. G., Fairbanks, L. A., Strickland, T., O'Connor, S. M., Rosenberg-Thompson, S., & Cummings, J.L. (2003). Frequency and characteristics of anxiety among patients with Alzheimer's disease and related dementias. *The Journal of Neuropsychiatry and Clinical Neurosciences*, 15, 180-186. doi: 10.1176/appi.neuropsych.15.2.180.

Price, J. L., & Morris, J. C. (1999). Tangles and plaques in nondemented aging and "preclinical" Alzheimer's disease. *Annals of neurlogy*, 45, 358-68. doi: 10.1002/1531-8249(199903)45:3<358::AID-ANA12>3.0.CO;2-X.

Riskind, J.H. & Alloy, L.B. (2006). Cognitive vulnerability to psychological disorders: Overview of theory, design, and methods. *Journal of Social and Clinical Psychology*, 25, 705-725. doi: 10.1521/jscp.2006.25.7.705.

Rosen, H.J., Gorno–Tempini, M.L., Goldman, W., Perry, R., Schuff, N., Weiner, M., Feiwell, R., Kramer, J. & Miller, B.L. (2002). Patterns of brain atrophy in frontotemporal dementia and semantic dementia. *Neurology*, 58,198-208. doi: 10.1212/WNL.58.2.198.

Rosenberg, P. B., & Lyketsos, C. (2008). Mild cognitive impairment: searching for the prodrome of Alzheimer's disease. *World Psychiatry*, 7, 72-78.

Royall, D. R. (1994). Precis of executive dyscontrol as a cause of problem behavior in dementia. *Experimental aging research*, 20, 73-94. doi: 10.1080/03610739408253955.

Sensi, S. V., Palitti, V.P., & Guagnano, M. T. (1993). Chronobiology in endocrinology. *Annali-istituto Superiore Di Sanita*, 29, 613-31.

Smith, M., & Buckwalter, K. (2005). Behaviors associated with dementia: Whether resisting care or exhibiting apathy, an older adult with dementia is attempting communication. Nurses and other caregivers must learn to 'hear' this language. *American Journal of Nursing*, 105, 40-52. doi: 10.1097/00000446-200507000-00028.

Van Cauter, E. (1990). Diurnal and ultradian rhythms in human endocrine function: a minireview. *Horm Research in Paediatrics*, 34, 45-53. doi: 10.1159/000181794.

Von Gunten, A., Pocnet, C., & Rossier, J. (2009). The impact of personality characteristics on the clinical expression in neurodegenerative disorders—A review. *Brain research bulletin*, 80, 179-191. doi: 10.1016/j.brainresbull.2009.07.004.

Weiten, W., Lloyd, M. A., Dunn D.S., & Hammer, E.Y. (2009). Coping Processes. In K. Makarewycz (Eds.) *Psychology applied to modern life: Adjustment in the 21st Century, Ninth Edition* (pp. 106 – 138). Belmont: Cengage Learning.

World Health Organization. (2012). *World Alzheimer Report 2012, A public health priority.* Available from: http: //whqlibdoc.who.int /publications/2012/9789241564458_eng.pd

Chapter 4: Classification of Behaviors in Dementia/NCD Based in Impairment in Theories Based Upon Information Processing Pathways

Introduction

This chapter is focused on the first theoretical construct of behaviors based upon Information Processing Theories (IPT). Behavioral categories emanating from IPT are the result of impairment in the functioning of information processing pathways. Such impairments can be a consequence of dysregulation of normal physiology, as is the case in delirium or structural decline, as is the case in cognitive impairments. In order to understand the implications of the impairment in information processing pathways on generation of behaviors, it is imperative to understand the role of these pathways in individuals with normal cognitive function.

Steps Involved in Information Processing

Arousal

Level of alertness or arousal may be defined as a state of wakefulness during which an individual is able to react to a stimulus (Thayer, 1989). It incorporates both physiological and psychological domains. Reticular activating system in the brain stem, autonomic nervous system and endocrine system are involved in the regulation of arousal. Arousal is involved in regulation of consciousness, attention and information processing (Thayer, 1989).

Attention

Attention is the factor that determines which mental representations of information are processed into memories, and how fast it is processed (Siegel, 2001). Components of attention that can affect the normal processing of information include selective attention, attention capacity, and sustained attention.

Selective attention refers to the concept that one can selectively choose which external or internal stimuli to process, and which to exclude, based upon its level of importance (Kietzman, Spring & Zubin, 1985). For instance, one can selectively focus attention to conversing with another individual in a room where several conversations are occurring at once. Attention capacity refers to the notion that one is only able to pay attention to a limited amount of input at a given moment. The number of different stimuli that are processed at once depends on how demanding each stimulus is on the overall system. Sustained attention is defined as the ability to consistently maintain a response during continuous thought processing (Siegel, 2001).

Information Processing

Atkinson and Shiffrin (1968) developed a stage model to explain the course of normal information processing. Atkinson and Shiffrin (1968) have titled this cascade *Information Processing Theory*. It is the most widely accepted approach to understanding the basis of cognition. "Cognition" involves mental processes such as awareness, judgment, perception, and reasoning for obtaining knowledge about information According to Atkinson and Shiffrin (1968) the main concepts of information processing include: input, sensory memory, short-term and long-term memory and output. "Memory" enables individuals to store and retrieve information through a series of steps and processes in the brain.

The first stage of the process is "input" of information (Atkinson & Shiffrin, 1968). This stage may be influenced by both external and internal stimuli. Sensation of external stimuli travels the peripheral sensory nervous system registering in the brain as information. The way in which information is internally organized and interpreted involves the processes of perception. This can occur both consciously and unconsciously (Siegel, 2001).

Sensory memory is the first stage of storing information (Atkinson & Shiffrin, 1968). External stimuli such as sounds, vision, tastes, and scents are all detected by the body's sensory receptor cells. Internal stimuli such as pain, touch, pressure, temperature, and vibration are also detected by the sensory receptor organs. All external and internal stimuli contain sources of energy. This energy is converted into electrical energy by the process of transduction. These electrical impulses in the brain form sensory memories. Sensory memories are very brief. Visual memories take approximately half a second to form while auditory memories take approximately three seconds (Nevid, 2012). The primary and secondary sensory areas of the cerebral cortex enable humans to form sensory memories.

The second stage of information processing is "short-term memory" (STM) (Atkinson & Shiffrin, 1968). STM involves consciously processing information. Thus, it is also referred to as "working memory." Encoding is a mechanism by which the information is processed through cortical and sub-cortical neuronal pathways to form "working memory". Steps which aid in encoding information into short-term memory include *rehearsal, chunking, imagery, schema activation, and pattern recognition.*

Rehearsal refers to repetition of incoming information. This allows for the information to remain in short-term memory for an extended period of time

(Nevid, 2012). Chunking refers to the idea that the brain can only process seven (plus or minus two) units of information at one given time (Miller, 1956). For instance, the letters "c" "t" and "a" are represented as three units of information when processed separately. However, when the letters are processed together as the word "cat", this constitutes only one unit of information. Combining letters together to form a word, as in this example, is referred to as *chunking* (Nevid, 2012). *Imagery* is the act of forming a mental image of a visual picture, sound, smell, taste, or touch sensation (Nevid, 2012). The sensory receptor organs are not stimulated in the process of imagery; only the brain is used (Kietzman, Zubin & Steinhauer, 1984). *Schema activation* involves pairing new knowledge to previously learned information about similar concepts and ideas. Schemas are networks of connected facts (Nevid, 2012). For example, a schema for zebras, penguins and Dalmatians would be black and white animals. These are also referred to as *"mental schemas"*. Mental schemas are the result of encoding of all sensory inputs to create an *"internal world model"* (Pezzulo et al., 2008). *Pattern recognition* involves comparing current patterns with previously identified patterns that are already stored in one's short or long-term memory (Nevid, 2012). In summary, the STM consists of any information an individual is consciously thinking of at that given moment in time. These memories are approximately twenty to thirty seconds in length (Nevid, 2012). All different types of memories (auditory and visual; short term and long term) are incorporated into the formation of cognitions or thoughts by the associational cortex. These are subsequently expressed through speech.

After the information has been handled through *primary* and *secondary sensory areas* of the cerebral cortex, subsequent process of encoding, storage, retrieval, and output of verbal, emotional, and motor behaviors occurs in the "association cortex". The integral components of associational cortex include the *limbic associationarea*, referring to the anterior-ventral part of the temporal lobe and parahippocampal gyrus, the *posterior association area*, referring to the junction of occipital, temporal and parietal lobes; and the *anterior associationarea*, referring to the prefrontal cortex. The prefrontal cortex is the major functional component of the brain responsible for STM.

For the sake of this article, we will refer to this entire structural and functional unit (*primary* and *secondary sensory areas* of the cerebral cortex, subsequent process of *encoding, storage, retrieval*, and *output of verbal, emotional,* and *motor behaviors* occurring in the *associationcortex*) as *information processing module* (IPM).

The information from all internal and external sources travels into the IPM and this is a two way process (Atkinson & Shiffrin, 1968). A two-way flow of information exists for the storage and retrieval of memories. Information is either voluntarily or involuntarily accessed through bottom-up or top-down processing. Bottom-up processing refers to the concept that information is processed from external stimuli to higher-order cognitive processes (Nevid, 2012). This process is also referred to as being stimulus-driven or data-driven. This type of processing often occurs automatically and without conscious awareness (Siegel, 2001). For example, reading a poem for the first time would involve bottom-up processing. In comparison, top-down processing involves using higher-order cognitive processes to give meaning to one's environment. The information being processed draws upon mental representations that are already stored in one's memory (Nevid, 2012). This process is also referred to as being conceptually-driven or theory-driven. Top-down processing places a higher working demand on the information processing system because it requires selective voluntary attention (Huitt, 2003). For instance, reading another individual's poor handwriting may require one to use top-down processing to identify any illegible words in the sentence.

The final step of the information-processing system is *output* (Atkinson & Shiffrin, 1968). The output response can be in the form of verbal (cognitive schema), emotions or motor behaviors. Information travel is also dynamic in nature in that the consequences of the interaction between the output cognitions, emotions, motor behaviors, and the environment are fed back through the input pathways for necessary and appropriate modifications to occur in the subsequent output. The two way flow of information and the dynamic interaction between the information flow and the environment is meant to be a sequential process.

Yerkes-Dodson Law

According to the Yerkes-Dodson Law, there is an intimate relationship between arousal, attention, information processing, and task performance (Yerkes & Dodson, 1908).

The level of alertness or arousal influences attention in a congruent manner. If the level of arousal is lethargic an individual becomes hypoattentive. If the level of arousal is hypervigilant an individual is distractible. In both instances, there is a negative impact on selective attention, attention capacity and sustained attention. In addition to the impact of arousal on attention, it also impacts on the speed with which the information is processed in the brain, information processing speed (IPS). Level of arousal and attention are together referred to as sensorium (Groth-Marnat, 2009). Sensorium has a congruent impact on IPS. Lethargy in arousal results in a decrease in IPS and a state of vigilance or hypervigilance will result in an increased IPS.

A schematic diagram which adequately represents the dynamic interaction amongst arousal, attention and IPM with subsequent output of higher cortical functions, cognitive schema, perceptions, emotions and motor behaviors is represented in Figure 1.

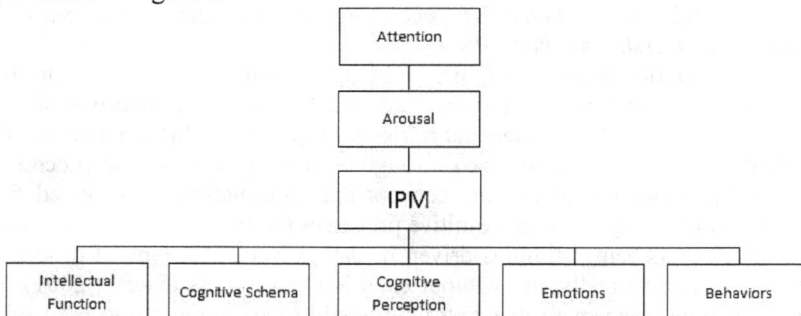

Figure 1 - Schematic Diagram of the Functional Model of the Human Brain (Luthra, 2012)

Figure 1 describes how arousal and attention (referred to as the sensorium) affect functioning of the IPM, which impacts a patient's intellectual function, cognitive schema, cognitive perception, emotions, and behaviors.

Information Processing in Pathological States

Impaired functioning of IPP can be a consequence of alterations in sensorium alone, impairment in functioning of IPM or a combination of both. Alterations in sensorium alone will impact on selectivity, capacity and sustenance of attention and the speed with which the information is traveling on the input arm of IPM. Bites of information being fed into and the speed with which it will travel on the input arm will influence how it is processed by IPM and subsequently impact on cognitive functioning. Changes in sensorium are the result of changes in the body's physiological status.

Dementia/NCD, results in breakdown of the neuronal circuitry involved in IPM thereby impairing its functional integrity. Impairment in functioning of the IPM, as a consequence of the disease processes in dementia/NCD, will thereby negatively impact cognitive functioning.

Similarly in preserved neurocircuitry, impairment in sensorium will impact negatively on the functional integrity of the IPM. If the neurocircuitry is impaired, as is the case in patients with dementia/NCDs, impairment in sensorium will result in an exponential impact on the functional integrity of IPM.

As is evident above, the impairment of the IPM will result in impairment in stimulus-driven and conceptually-driven flow of information. This will result in cognitive difficulties in memory and other higher cortical functions including language, visuo-spatial, executive functioning, and praxis. Severity of the impairment of the IPM is determined by the severity and type of dementia/NCD. In the moderate to advanced stages of dementia/NCD, impairment in working memories, as a consequence of impaired encoding processes, will result in generation of distorted cognitive schema and cognitive perceptions. Subsequent generation of emotions and behaviors is determined by these distorted schema and perceptions. The distortions of cognitive schema and perceptions will ultimately manifest as behaviors of the disorganised and misidentification type.

Disorganised Behaviors

Criteria and format put forth by Davis, Buckwalter and Burgio (1997) will be used structure the behavioral category.

Items in the Disorganized Behavior Category Include

- Appearing "vacant" or "blank" in facial expressions and mental lethargy;
- Disorganized thinking, unintelligible/garbled speech
- Rapid shifts in or incongruence of emotional states
- Inappropriate mixing of food or clothing and layering, smearing fecal matter, playing in the toilet bowl or global functional decline

- Playing with things in the air, responding to auditory hallucinations, picking things from the body or furniture

Purpose of the Measure or "Meaning of Behavior"

- Recognition of behaviors in this category is to make the health care givers and providers aware of the superimposed "muddled" or "confused" states occurring in patients with underlying dementia/NCDs. It is to make clinicians aware of the emergence of an *organic mental syndrome (OMS)* in the patient. OMS is defined as a change in arousal, cognition, mentation or functioning as a consequence of a physiological dysregulation from any etiology (Purdie, Honigman & Rosen, 1981). It is outside the scope of this article to argue the merits of this diagnostic category. Suffice it to say, not all patients who exhibit OMS will go on to develop a full spectrum delirium syndrome. A significant majority of patients only demonstrate a singular change in any of these four domains.
- Health care professionals, who work intimately with patients with dementia/NCDs, are able to recognise subtle changes in individual patients' level of alertness, cognitive and functional abilities from their respective baseline. It is not uncommon to hear the staff mention that "Mr. Smith is more confused of late" or "there is something different about Mrs. Smith today".
- Identification of the behaviors in this category is to alert health care professionals to changes in underlying physiological status of the patients from baseline.
- In these situations, changes in physiological status are often the result of dysregulation in the *modifiable* variables. *Modifiable* variables are inclusive of changes in bowels habits, inadequate bladder emptying, changes in hearing due to wax or foreign objects, changes in vision changes due to loss of vision aids or unkempt lens, gum and dentition, pain, medication side effects and circadian rhythm changes. Infections of the urinary and respiratory tracts and fluid balance shifts are contributory as wells. If clinically indicated, the list of variables can be expanded to include the exhaustive list used to work up a case of delirium.
- The initial approach to treatment of behaviors in this category is to identify and rectify the underlying etiology responsible for the physiological change from baseline. Next steps include providing adequate supportive care.
- Supportive care is inclusive of but not exhaustive to include hydration, nutrition, skin care, fall prevention, safe swallowing, diminishing stimulation, repeated attempts to re-orient the patient with judicious use of pharmacological interventions.
- The clinicians should remain vigilant to the progression of the clinical condition to a full blown delirium. If a diagnosis of delirium is confirm, best practice guidelines are in place for managing this clinical condition.

Specification of the "Construct" of the Category

The principal dysregulation underlying the genesis of disorganized behaviors is a "presumed disconnectedness" of information processing at many different levels involving the cortex, sub-cortex, midbrain, brain stem and the cerebellum; a phenomenon of impaired IPS.

For disorganized behaviors to occur there has to be a change in the patient's physiological status from baseline status. Physiological dysregulation will impact on arousal with congruent changes in attention, combined known as "sensorium". Changes in sensorium result in the impairment of the sequential organization of information processing cascade; giving way to fragmentation of the process at many different levels of the brain and as noted above. This fragmentation in information processing cannot be successfully integrated by a patient into a cohesive message; therefore, the level of severity of impairment in sensorium and subsequent breakdown in information flow will give way to a hierarchy of behavioral symptoms.

Mild impairment in sensorium may result in the interruption of information transfer along the input pathways. The information is unable to be registered as sensory memory and subsequently unavailable for the process of encoding. The patient will present themselves as appearing perplexed, vague, or bewildered. This will be expressed through facial expressions as appearing "vacant" or "blank".

Moderate levels in impairment of sensorium may result in interruption of the encoding process. This degree of impairment will result in disruption in formation of thought and its expression through speech. Disorganized thinking, unintelligible, or garbled speech are examples of this stage of impairment.

As the level of severity in impairment of sensorium reaches severe proportions, it impacts on the associational cortex and subsequently output pathways. As a result, there is reduction in expression of symptoms through thoughts and speech, but more reduction occurs through emotional and motor behaviors. Examples of expression through emotions include rapid shifts in emotional states or incongruence in emotional states. Examples of expression through motor behaviors include inappropriate mixing of food or clothing and layering of clothing, smearing fecal matter, playing in toilet bowl or a global decline in functioning.

The ultimate breakdown of the functional integrity of IPM may result in patients experiencing perceptual abnormalities in the absence of obvious stimuli. Examples of this include playing with things in the air, responding to auditory hallucinations, or picking things off the body or furniture

Misidentification Behaviors

Criteria and format put forth by Davis, Buckwalter and Burgio (1997) were used to structure the misidentification behavior category.

Items in the Misidentification Behavior Category Include

- Misidentification of persons, places, objects

- Misidentification of sounds, smells, tastes or touch
- Misidentification of events or occurrences
- Misperception or interpretation of comments or behaviors of others

Purpose of the Measure or "Meaning of Behavior"

- Recognition of behaviors in this category assists health care givers (CG) and care provider's (CP) awareness of "paranoid" states existing in patients with dementia/NCD. Misidentification of "persons" and "places" will often take the form of identifying another patient as the spouse or the facility as the home.
- Recognition of the behaviors in this category should alert CG or CP to the probability of their verbal and non-verbal interactions with the patient to be misunderstood.
- Presence of symptoms in this behavioral category should alert staff to take the needed extra time to explain everything in detail, in a very simple manner.
- At the first indication of being misconstrued, a change in care plan needs to be effected to reflect all interactions with the patient to be done in pairs, documenting all interactions in detail.

Specification of the "Construct" of the Category

The principle dysregulation underlying the genesis of misidentification behaviors is an alteration in the relationship between self and other persons, places, objects, events or their comments or behaviors in the presence of a clear sensorium (Silva et al., 2000).

In existing literature, this behavioral category is widely known as Delusional Misidentification Syndromes (DMS). DMS is a clinical condition in which patients develop fixed beliefs based upon misidentification of existing stimuli. Common stimuli are often in the form of persons, places, objects, and events. These stimuli are often of great personal importance to the patient. DMS is a separate clinical entity from hallucinations whereby patients will experience a perception in the absence of a stimulus. Tamam et al. (2003) found the incidence of DMS in the range of 1.3 to 4.1% in all psychiatric inpatients and rates as high as 15% in inpatients with a diagnosis of schizophrenia. Harwood et al. (1999) have found the rates to be as high as 10% in patients with dementia/NCD of Alzheimer type (DAT). Ballard et al. (1999) have reported a higher incidence of DMS in patients with Lewy Body Dementia/NCD (LBD) in comparison to DAT.

There is absence of consensus on the pattern of cognitive impairment in patients experiencing DMS (Joseph, 1986; Feinberg & Shapiro, 1989; Weinstein & Burnham, 1991). Most data, however, seems to support the combined presence of impairment in memory, executive, and visuo-spatial functions as a requisite for emergence of DMS (Alexander, Stuss & Benson, 1979; Staton, Brumback & Wilson, 1982). Feinberg & Roane (2005) propose the basis of DMS as an altered sense of relatedness between self and other persons, places, objects and events. Staton, Brumback & Wilson (1982) proposed a degree of disconnectedness occurs at the level of encoding of new information into working memory. There is dehiscence between two of the steps involved in the encoding process and these steps are schema activation and pattern recognition. As a consequence, the pairing of new and familiar information does not occur in the usual manner and it leads to an altered sense of relatedness between self and the persons, places, objects, and events.

Neurophysiological markers in the form of Event Related Potentials (ERP) are used to establish functional integrity of neuronal circuitry (Fabiani Gratton & Coles, 2000). P300 ERP represents the functional integrity of the neuronal pathways involved in encoding of *working memory*. Patients with DMS show substantially attenuated amplitude of P300 at F4, P3, and Pz abductions in comparison to healthy controls (Papageorgiou et al., 2002). These findings support the theoretical constructs regarding the disconnectedness at the level of encoding of new information put forth by Staton, Brumback & Wilson (1982).

As mentioned above, the occurrence of misidentified behaviors results from the improper processing of sensory stimuli. Visual stimuli are divided into "facial" and "non-facial" (referring to everything in the environment except faces) stimuli as a way to better understand the pathology in misidentification behaviors (Ellis et al., 1993). There can be "mis" or "over" identification with facial and non-facial stimuli in the pathological states (Mori et al., 2000). Only misidentification occurs with auditory, gustatory, tactile, or olfactory stimuli in the pathological states. There is no evidence of "over" identification of any of these perceptions in pathological states.

Example of misidentification of facial stimulus involves the patient accusing a family member of looking and acting like their loved one but being an imposter, such as in Capgras syndrome (Silva et al., 2000). Example of misidentification of non-facial stimuli, such as their environment, involves a patient wanting to "go home" when they are already in their home. The patient is misidentifying the environment as someone else's home. Over-identification of facial stimulus involves a patient labelling another patient on the floor as the spouse and attempting to be intimate with them. Over-identification of non-facial stimuli involves a patient labelling the hospital or the LTCF as their home and all the patients or residents are intruders or boarders and not paying their fair share of rent (Fregoli Syndrome). This leads to further conflicts between and amongst the patients or residents.

Example of misidentifying auditory stimulus involves a patient accusing the caregiver or medical/nursing provider of yelling or screaming at even though the conversation took place at a normal volume of speech. Another example of misidentifying auditory stimulus involves a patient listening to the air flow from the vent above his bed and asking the staff to turn of the water before he drowns. In this case, the air gushing out is being perceived as a tap running and potentially flooding the room.

Example of misidentifying tactile stimulus involves a patient allegedly accusing the caregiver or provider of acts of physical aggression during care. Usual handling of the patient in transfers with the help of mechanical lifts, its ebbs and flows, is misinterpreted by the patient as acts of physical aggression. An example of misidentifying olfactory stimulus involves a patient panicking, believing the building is on fire after they smell smoke from a toaster oven. An example of patient misidentifying gustatory stimulus involves the patient allegedly accusing the nurse of poisoning them on the basis of the bitter taste of the medicine.

An example of misidentification of events or occurrences may include a patient labelling a group activity involving crafts as a celebration of their birthday. Another example could include a patient labelling a medical emergency on the ward and a team response to "code blue" as an act of terrorism resulting in chaos on the unit.

An example of misinterpretation by the patient is of conversation amongst staff or patients as, "they are talking about me or making fun of me". Continued misinterpretation of the conversation could lead to the patient construing "they are plotting to harm me". Along the same lines a patient might misconstrue other patient behavior as threatening or intimidating. As an example, they could see the patient carrying a book in their hand and walking towards them as an overt act of aggression.

Conclusions

Pathological changes in information processing, due to varied etiologies, results in cognitive impairment of varying severity. According to DSM-IV-TR, impairment in working memory along with one other higher cortical function along with a decline in function is required to be diagnosed with dementia/NCD.

There are several steps involved in the encoding process to form working memory. Integrity of this process is essential in generation of thoughts or cognitions. Cognitions generate emotions with subsequent emergence of congruent behaviors. In all patients with dementia/NCD, irrespective of etiology, the initial impairment occurs in encoding of working memories. Any of the steps involved in encoding process (rehearsal, chunking, imagery, schema activation and pattern recognition) can be impaired in patients with dementia/NCDs. Severity of the impairment in encoding process is determined by the advancement and stage of dementia/NCD process. In the moderate to advanced stages of dementia/NCD, the encoding process will be congruently impaired with emergence of impaired working memories. These working memories emerging from such an impaired encoding process, as well as impairment in top-down or bottom-up flow of information will result in generation of distorted cognitive schema and cognitive perceptions. These lead to emergence of congruent emotions and behaviors.

Hence, the primary pathophysiology determining the *Quality* of behaviors, irrespective of etiology, under several of the identified Behavioral categories, is the generation of distorted cognitive schema and cognitive perceptions. Examples of behaviors emanating as a result of this pathophysiology are MiB, GDB, subtypes of VB, FTB and subtypes of SB).

Disorganized behaviors are the result of an alteration in the physiological status of the patient which results in changes in their sensorium. Change in sensorium also causes a change in IPS. Impaired information processing pathways in patients with dementia/NCD are further compromised and debilitated by these added physiological changes. These changes result in breakdown in the sequential organization of information to a fragmented process. Severity of impairment will give rise to hierarchy of symptoms and as described in the section under disorganized behaviors.

Behaviors based in misidentification are the result of a specific breakdown in schema identification and pattern recognition, two final steps, of the encoding process. This will result in the failure of usual pairing of the old and new information with an altered sense of relatedness between self and persons, places, objects and events.

References

Alexander, M. P., Stuss, D. T., & Benson, D. F. (1979). Capgras syndrome: A reduplicative phenomenon. *Neurology*, 29, 334-339. doi: 10.1212/WNL.29.3.334.

Atkinson, R. C., & Shiffrin, R. M. (1968). Human Memory: A Proposed System and its Control Processes. In G. H. Bower, & J. T. Spence, *Psychology of Learning and Motivation: Advances in Research and Theory*, volume 2. (pp. 89-196). New York: Academic Press Inc.

Ballard, C., Holmes, C., McKeith, I., Neill, D., O'Brien, J., Cairns, N., Lantos, P., Perry, E., Ince, P., & Perry, R. (1999). Psychiatric morbidity in dementia with Lewy bodies: a prospective clinical and neuropathological comparative study with Alzheimer's disease. *American Journal of Psychiatry*, 156, 1039-1045.

Davis, L. L., Buckwalter, K., & Burgio, L. D. (1997). Measuring problem behaviors in dementia: developing a methodological agenda. *Advances in Nursing Science*, 20, 40-55.

Ellis, H. D., de Pauw, K. W., Christodoulou, G. N., Papageorgiou, L., Milne, A. B., & Joseph, A. B. (1993). Responses to facial and non-facial stimuli presented tachistoscopically in either or both visual fields by patients with the Capgras delusion and paranoid schizophrenics. *Journal of Neurology, Neurosurgery, and Psychiatry*, 56, 215-219. doi: 10.1136/jnnp.56.2.215.

Fabiani, M., Gratton, G., & Coles, M. (2000). Event-related potentials: methods, theory, and applications. In J. Cacioppo, L. Tassinary, & G. Bernston (Eds.), *Handbook of Psychophysiology*. (pp. 53-84). New York: Cambridge University Press.

Feinberg, T. E., & Roane, D. M. (2005). Delusional misidentification. *Psychiatric Clinics of North America*, 28, 665-683. doi: 10.1016/j.psc.2005.05.002.

Feinberg, T. E., & Shapiro, R. M. (1989). Misidentification-reduplication and the right hemisphere. *Neuropsychiatry, Neuropsychology, & Behavioral Neurology*, 2, 39-48. doi: 10.1093/acprof:oso/9780195173413.003.0008.

Groth-Marnat, G. (2009). Mental Status Examination. In The Assessment Interview, (Eds.) *Handbook of psychological assessment*, 4th edition. (pp. 82 – 83) Hoboken: Wiley.

Harwood, D., Barker, W. W., Ownby, R. L., & Duara, R. (1999). Prevalence and correlates of Capgras syndrome in Alzheimer's disease. *International Journal of Geriatric Psychiatry*, 14, 415-20. doi: 10.1002/(SICI)1099-1166(199906)14:6<415::AID-GPS929>3.0.CO;2-3.

Huitt, W. (2003). *The Information Processing Approach to Cognition*. Available from: http://www.edpsycinteractive.org/topics/cognition/infoproc.html

Joseph, A. B. (1986). Focal central nervous system abnormalities in patients with misidentification syndromes. *Bibliotheca Psychiatrica*, 164, 68-79.

Kietzman, M. L., Zubin, J., & Steinhauer, S. R. (1984). Information Processing in Psychopathology. In V. Sarris, & A. Parducci (Eds.), *Perspectives in Psychological Experimentation: Towards the Year 2000*. (pp. 291-309). Hillsdale: Erlbaum.

Kietzman, M., Spring, B., & Zubin, J. (1985). Perception, cognition, and information processing. In H. I. Kaplin, & B. Sadock (Eds.), *Comprehensive textbook of psychiatry (4th ed.)* (pp. 157-178). Baltimore: Williams and Wilkins.

Miller, G. A. (1956). The magical number seven plus or minus two: some limits on our capacity for processing information. *The Psychological Review*, 63, 81-97. doi: 10.1037/h0043158.

Mori, E. et al. (2000). Visuoperceptual impairment in dementia with Lewy bodies. *Archives of neurology*, 4, 489-493. doi: 10.1001/archneur. 57.4.489.

Nevid, J.S. (2012). *Psychology: Concepts and Applications Third Edition*. Belmont: Wadsworth Cengage Learning.

Papageorgiou, C., Lykouras, L., Ventouras, E., Uzunoglu, N., & Christodoulou, G. N. (2002). Abnormal P300 in a case of delusional misidentification with coinciding Capgras and Frégoli symptoms. *Progress in Neuropsychopharmacology and Biological Psychiatry*, 26, 805-810. doi: 10.1016/S0278-5846(01)00293-7.

Pezzulo, G., Butz, M. V., Castelfranchi, C., & Falcone, R. (Eds.). (2008). *The challenge of anticipation: A unifying framework for the analysis and design of artificial cognitive systems* (Vol. 5225). New York: Springer-Verlag Incorporated.

Purdie, F. R., Honigman, B., & Rosen, P. (1981). Acute organic brain syndrome: a review of 100 cases. *Annals of Emergency Medicine*, 9, 455-461. doi: 10.1016/S0196-0644(81)80276-4.

Siegel, D. J. (2001). Memory: an overview, with emphasis on developmental, interpersonal, and neurobiological aspects. *Journal of the American Academy of Child Adolescent & Psychiatry*, 40, 997-1011. doi: 10.1097/00004583-200109000-00008.

Silva, J. A., Leong, G. B., Weinstock, R., & Ruiz-Sweeney, M. (2000). Delusional misidentification and aggression in Alzheimer's disease. *Journal of Forensic Sciences*, 46, 581-585.

Staton, R. D., Brumback, R. A., & Wilson, H. (1982). Reduplicative paramnesia: a disconnection syndrome of memory. *Cortex*, 18, 23-35. doi: 10.1093/neucas/4.3.255-o.

Tamam, L., Karatas, G., Zeren, T., & Ozpoyraz, N. (2003). The prevalence of Capgras syndrome in a university hospital setting. *Acta Neuropsychiatrica*, 15, 290-295. doi: 10.1034/j.1601-5215.2003. 00039.x.

Thayer, R. E. (1989). The biopsychology of mood and arousal. In (Ed.), *Arousal: A basic element for mood and behavior.* pp. 46 – 66. Oxford: University Press on Demand.

Weinstein, E. A., & Burnham, D. L. (1991). Reduplication and the syndrome of Capgras. *Psychiatry*, 54, 78-88.

Yerkes, R.M., & Dodson, J.D. (1908). The relationship of strength of stimulus to rapidity of habit formation. *Journal of Comparative Neurology and Psychology*, 18, 459-482.

Chapter 5: Classification of Behaviors in Dementia/NCD Based in "Motivational" and "Needs Based" Theories

Introduction

This paper is focused on the second theoretical construct of behaviors based upon "motivational" and "needs based" theories. Behavioral categories emanating from "motivational" and "needs based" theories are the result of impairment in the motivational circuits in the brain and which is a direct consequence of cognitive impairment; irrespective of the etiology. In order to understand the implications of the impairment of the motivational circuits on generation of behaviors, it is imperative to understand the structure and function of motivational circuits in individuals with normal cognitive function.

Motivational and Needs Based Theories

One of the first models for understanding the presence of behaviors in dementia/NCD was based in *unmet needs* (Algase et al.,1996). It was titled "unmet needs based" behaviors in patients with dementia/NCDs (Algase et al.,1996). This was later modified by Kovach et al. (2005) and titled *Need-Driven Dementia/NCD-Compromised Behavior* (C-NDB). C-NDB posits *Background, Proximal, Personal, Care,* and *Contextual factors* coalesce and interact amongst each other in the following manner; *Background* and *Proximal* factors interact with each other to generate unmet needs which give rise to primary behaviors. If these behaviors lead to fulfillment of the underlying needs it will result in settling down of the generated behaviors. If the needs remain unmet, "primary unmet needs" behaviors will interact with *Personal, Care,* and *Contextual* factors to generate "secondary" needs based behaviors (Kovach et al., 2005).

An alternative body of literature in behavioral psychology addresses the area of motivation and needs and the dynamic interaction between the two variables. Motivation has its origins from the Latin term *movere*, meaning "to move". Consensus definition of motivation is the force acting on or within an individual which results in arousal, direction, and persistence of goal-directed, voluntary effort. While needs are created by physiological or psychological deficiencies or imbalances (Kovach et al., 2005), such a deficiency becomes the basis for drives. "Drives", which are also referred to as motives, propel the individual to meet and satisfy their needs in order to achieve their goal. Incentives alleviate needs thereby lessening the intensity of drives. Therefore, needs and motivation coexist.

Motivational theories provide the understanding of "why" and "how" of human behavior; with several motivational theories have been put forth. Motivational theories can be broadly classified into two main subtypes: content and process theories of motivation. Content (or Needs) theories of motivation help us understand the "what" and "why" of human behavior. Whereas, process (or Cognitive) theories of motivation help us to understand the "how to" motivate human behavior.

Content theories deal with prioritizing an individual's needs from "basic" to "higher" level needs. Content theories deal with the factors and variables which help us understand "what" motivates an individual and "why" they occur. *Maslow's Hierarchy of Needs theory* was the first of the content theories of motivation (Maslow, 1943). Extensions and modifications of Maslow's *Hierarchy of Needs* theory include Herzberg's (1959) *Motivation-Hygiene theory* (Herzberg, Mausner & Snyderman, 1959) and McClelland's (1967) *Learned Needs theories*. Maslow's *Hierarchy of Needs theory* will be used for discussion purposes in this article.

Content (or Need) theories of motivation identify a hierarchy of needs from "basic" to "higher" levels. According to Maslow's Hierarchy of needs theory (1943), the ascending level of hierarchy consists of physiological, such as hunger, thirst, sex, rest, social, and mental stimulation; security, such as physical safety and psychological security; belongingness, such as affiliation, acceptance, being a part of something or striving for something; esteem, such as respect from others, self-respect, and recognition; and self-actualization, such as reaching your maximum potential and doing your best. Fulfillment of esteem and self-actualization needs require the highest level of intellectual functioning in order to generate complex cognitive schemas through interaction between an individual and their environment. Patients with dementia/NCDs are incapable of such a high level of intellectual functioning. Physiological, security and belongingness needs are more innate and basic. It is these needs that are preserved even with significant loss in intellectual function, as happens in patients with moderate to advanced stages of dementia/NCD (Hancock et al., 2006).

Process, or cognitive, theories of motivation deal with "how" to motivate individuals. Major process theories include *Expectancy theory* (Vroom, 1964), *Goal-Setting theory* (Locke et al., 1981), and *Reinforcement theory* (Skinner, 1953). The majority of the literature regarding process theories is set in the context of human behavior in organizational settings. This research is based upon the premise of an individual functioning at the highest level of their intellectual abilities, that which is compatible with occupational functioning. Such a high level of occupational functioning is only feasible in the absence of any intellectual or cognitive impairment. Hence, there is no applicability of process theories to the dementia/NCD population.

Overview of Motivational Circuitry

Motivational circuitry (MC) in the brain regulates the degree of motivational energy or drives in an individual propelling them to meet their needs. Motivation circuitry processes information via the "input" arm of the circuitry. This includes information on the discrepancy between the internal state of the individual and their external environment in order to determine the most appropriate behavioral "output" to fulfill the identified needs. The MC consists of a Primary Motivation Circuit (PMC) which is supported by Secondary Motivational Circuits (SMC). PMC consists of the cortico-straital-thalamic-cortical pathways. These pathways originate in the Prefrontal cortex and travel via the straitum and the thalamus ending up back in the prefrontal cortex. These pathways are primarily innervated by dopaminergic fibers. The principle function of these pathways is to select motivational drives and prioritize decision making for a specific behavioral action. There may be several needs identified at any given point in time and the role of these pathways is to prioritize as to which of the needs will be fulfilled first. SMC consist of the following:

I.   Glutaminergic fibers originating in the prefrontal cortex (PFC), travelling via the amygdala (A), hippocampus (H), and ventral globus pallidus (VGP) to end up in nucleus accumbens (NA). These circuits are responsible for transferring affective and contextual memory information to the NA.

II.   Gabaminergic fibers originate in NA and travel via the Ventral Tegmental Area (VTA), VGP, and Thalamus ending up in the Prefrontal cortex. These circuits carry the information on the "selected motivation drives" to the prefrontal cortex.

III. Dopaminergic fibers in the form of medial forebrain bundle (MFB) and mesolimbic pathways (MLP); the MFB consists of axons arising in the basal olfactory regions and the septal nuclei to form the main dopaminergic pathways. MFB relays information from VTA to NA. MLP are also primarily dopaminergic fibers which originate in VTA and travel via NA, Amygdala onto medial PFC. These pathways are responsible for identification of novel stimuli in the environment which trigger needs and modulation of motivational drives into behavioral actions.

Model of Relationship between Needs and Motivation

Common view assumes that all goal pursuits are governed by a conscious, intentional, planning process and require relative preservation of executive function (Deci & Ryan, 2000). Whereas this may be true for goal pursuits in an organizational setting, recent developments in social psychology suggests that much of the social goal directed behavior, governing satiation of belongingness needs, occurs largely in an automatic way and without any involvement of conscious intent (Custers & Aarts, 2010). This hypothesis has been proven by creation of an artificial animal (an animat) to generate goal directed behaviors. This model functions at a very simplistic level; the structural format of the "animat" consists of sensory-motor loops capable of carrying structured stimulus, details of metric spatial information, and an adaptive training algorithm. The animat's circuit has nowhere near the complexity of the human brain. Such an animat was capable of learning associations between sensory inputs and motor outputs and adapt accordingly to generate new goal directed behaviors. There is sufficient evidence to support the notion that individual neuronal networks possess the property of synaptic plasticity and behavioral adaptation well into the late stages of dementia/NCD (Greenwood, 2007). Hence, it is reasonable to propose that even with progressive cognitive impairment and well into the late stages of the disease, the brain maintains its ability to generate socially determined goal directed behaviors.

Motivational theories have attempted to understand how living organisms act when they perceive a discrepancy between themselves and their environment. Control theories of motivation are centered on the principle of reduction of goal-environment discrepancies. According to this subset of theories, any time an organism perceives a discrepancy in their milieu (i.e. interaction between the organism and the environment) some action needs to be taken to reduce the discrepancy (Gibson, 1997). Gibson (1997), using an ecological approach to psychology, defined the concept of "affordances", referring to the "action of possibilities that various objects offer to an organism, situated in that environment." The action possibilities offered by an environment to an organism acting in it are perceived by the organisms as opportunities in that environment to achieve their specific behavioral results. These generated behaviors are responsible for satiation of belongingness needs.

The perceived discrepancy between an organism's internal state and a stimulus in their environment forms the basis for triggering a physiological or psychological deficiency. This deficiency leads to identification of a specific need. The relevant information of the identified need travels via the SMC. This relevant information consists of sensory, affective, and contextual memory and hormonal/homeostatic processes associated with the identified need. Two important steps in encoding of working memory are schema activation and pattern recognition (Anderson, 1977). The purpose of both of these steps is to pair the incoming information with the stored information in order to provide context and meaning to the new information (Anderson, 1977). Goal-representations or "mental schemas" are the result of encoding of all sensory inputs to create an "internal world model" (Pezzulo et al., 2008). Hence, any time there is a perceived discrepancy between the organism and its environment, there is activation of these mental schemas (Pezzulo et al., 2008). The information on the activated mental schemas is relayed to the PMC via the SMC. PMC are responsible for selection of specific motivational drives and prioritizing decision making on specific behavioral actions. These drives and behavioral actions lead to a reduction in the identified discrepancy with resulting satisfaction or satiation of the need. This behavioral output is governed by the *ideomotor principle*; according to this principle, actions are controlled bi-directionally through the results they produce (Pezzulo et al., 2008).

Summary of Circuit and Function

A stimulus in the environment may trigger a physiological or a psychological deficiency or it may be triggered by an internal stimulus. Either of these stimuli will generate a need which requires fulfillment. These needs tend be physiological, security, or belongingness in nature in patients with even advanced stages of dementia/NCD. Relevant sensory, affective, contextual memory and hormonal/homeostatic information is carried by SMC to the PMC. PMC is responsible for selection of motivational drive and prioritizing decision making to produce a specific behavioral action. This will lead to satisfaction or satiation with the release of the needs.

Motivational circuits are impacted in a variety of disease states including dementia/NCDs. In some type of dementia/NCDs, such as frontal lobe dementia/NCDs, these circuits may be affected at an earlier stage in the course of the disease but invariably are affected in the latter stages of all dementia/NCDs, irrespective of the etiology. Motivational energy can be either increased or decreased in disease states such as dementia/NCD. Accordingly, four types of behaviors can be described on the basis of motivational and needs based theories.

Behavioral Classification

Four behavioral categories emanating from motivational and needs based theories are:

    I.   Apathy behavior
    II.   Goal-directed behaviors
    III.   Motor behaviors
    IV.   Importuning behaviors

Apathy Behaviors

Items in the Category Include:

- Indifference and lack of concern re: self and environment
- Lack of self-initiation, low social engagement (inter-personal interactions; and milieu structure) and poor persistence
- Emotional indifference and acknowledgement of lack of emotional remorse

Purpose of the Measure or "Meaning of the Behavior"

- "Needs" identification is the consequence of a discrepancy between an organism's internal state and a stimulus in their immediate environment. Once the need has been identified, its fulfilment requires activation of motivational forces. These forces propel the individual to satiate the "need" thereby reducing the "need". Behaviors in this category are the result of diminished or absence of motivational drives due to the disease state of dementia/NCD.

- Lower motivational drives can impact on cognitions, behaviors and/or the concomitant emotions. "Indifference or lack of concern re; self or milieu" is the result of the impact of diminished motivational drives on cognitions. "Lack of initiation and poor persistence" are the result of the impact of diminished motivational drives on behaviors. "Emotional indifference and acknowledgement of lack of remorse" are the result of impact of diminished motivational drives on emotions.
- Recognition of behaviors in this category is to make care givers (CG) or care providers (CP) aware of the "lazy" states in patients with dementia/NCD. Though sounding pejorative, the term "lazy" is being used to dispel that very connotation attached to these behaviors by CG or CP.
- The patients with these behaviors require significant cuing and encouragement to initiate any activity, no matter how trivial the task. If and once the patients are seen to be engaged, they will cease activity and are unable to persist with the initiated tasks. Patients may tend to leave tasks incomplete despite repeated reminders. This tends to frustrate the CG and CP. Despite overt emotional expressions of this frustration, there is little to no acknowledgement of lack of emotional remorse, through verbal or non-verbal communication, being exhibited by the patient. If any expression is expressed it is more of indifference. This, further, aggravates the CG or CP thus potentially creating an unhealthy dynamic such that even less is accomplished of any intended task.
- Being aware of the symptoms in this category is to be informed of the unintentional or non-malicious intent underlying these behaviors. This should lead to increased tolerance and in development of care plans which reflect a graduated approach to tasks being accomplished.

Specification of the Construct of the Category

The principle dysregulation underlying the genesis of these behaviors is a varying degree of reduction in motivational drives. Clinically, patients experiencing apathy present slowed down in their thinking, emotions and activities.

Apathy is prevalent in up to 92% of all persons with a severe cognitive impairment (Mega et al., 1996). There is much debate on whether apathy should be considered a symptom or a syndrome. Further, there is a lack of consensus on criteria for diagnosing apathy (Starkstein & Leentjens, 2008). It is outside the scope of this article to explore the evolution of this concept since its inception by Greek philosophers of the "School of Stoic" over 2000 years ago; although they did coin the term "apathes"; meaning "loss of passion" (Starkstein & Leentjens, 2008). Many researchers have attempted to put forth a clinical presentation of this clinical condition. Landes et al. (2001), described apathy as, "a loss of motivation that manifests in behaviors such as diminished initiation, poor persistence, lack of interest, indifference, low social engagement, blunted emotional response, and lack of insight". Clarke et al. (2008) further conceptualized apathy as "the absence of responsiveness to stimuli as demonstrated by a lack of self-initiated action, lack of concern, and emotional indifference". The application of the construct of apathy for this article is in keeping with the criteria proposed by

Marin and Wilkosz (2005). According to Marin and Wilkosz (2005), apathy is a construct of diminished or absent, in severe forms, of motivational forces. Diminished motivational forces will impact on two domains: thinking or cognitions and activities. Emotional concomitants of these cognitions or activities may or may not be a part of the construct, depending on varied points of view (Marin and Wilkosz, 2005). Starkstein & Leentjens (2008) put forth criteria which appear to have a reasonably broad acceptance and those criteria are as follows:

I.   Diminished Goal Directed Cognition (GDC)
   •   Lack of motivation in learning new things or in new experiences
   •   Lack of concerns about one's personal problems
II.   Diminished Goal Directed Activities (GDA)
   •   Lack of energy or effort to perform everyday activities.
   •   Dependency on prompts from others to structure everyday activities
III. Diminished emotional concomitants of GDC and GDA
   •   Unchanging or flat affect (decrease in range of affect expressed)
   •   Lack of emotional responsiveness to positive and negative events.

Lower level of motivation results in a diminished level of interest in interacting with the environment and less of an individual's ability to recognize a deficiency between their internal state and the environment. The absence of identification of a need results in a reduction of goal directed cognitions, and subsequently activities.

Varying degrees of motivational decline can occur in disease states. A mildly diminished level of motivation will lead to a decrease in GDC and this will present itself as "indifference and lack of concern re; self or environment". A further decrease in motivational forces will lead to decrease in GDA and present itself as lack of self-initiation, low social engagement (both in interpersonal interactions and interactions with the milieu) and poor persistence. Diminished emotional concomitants to GDC and GDA will present in the form of emotional indifference and acknowledgement of lack of emotional remorse. It is outside the scope of this paper to review the difference between major depression and apathy. However, major depression is at the top of the list of differentials to be considered prior to diagnosing apathy.

Goal Directed Behaviors

Items in this Category Include:

   •   Goal directed cognitions such as "I am going home today, I am going to the bank, I am getting married today, where can I pay my bills"
   •   Goal directed activities (rummaging, rifling or emptying drawers; stripping clothes, rearranging furniture or fixing items in milieu; stripping bedding or pulling curtains/fixtures on the walls; bed/chair exiting or exit seeking
   •   Intrusiveness or purposeful wandering (seemingly driven, "on the go")

Purpose of the Measure or "Meaning of the Behavior"

- Recognition of behaviors in this category is to ensure care givers (CG) or care providers (CP) are aware of the "busy beaver" like state in patients with dementia/NCD. These patients tend to be very persistent with their demands and actions thereby creating a very high energy environment.

- When a patient perceives a discrepancy between their internal state and a stimulus in their milieu, it forms the basis of triggering a "need" which requires fulfilment. Motivational forces propel the patient to satiate these "needs". The degree of activation of motivational forces generated will determine whether the needs are expressed as "thoughts" or "action". Behaviors in this category are the result of heightened motivational drives due to the disease state of dementia/NCD.

- The specific need requiring fulfilment by these behaviors is that of "belongingness". The "belongingness" need encompasses being affiliated or accepted by ones milieu or environment, working towards and meeting one's obligations and responsibilities in order to be a part of larger society or milieu. Hence, the locus of control for these needs underlying the genesis of GDC or GDA tends to be external to the patient and the triggers are present in their immediate external environment.

- If the "busy" states involve thinking and as is the case in these set of behaviors, patients are repeatedly coming up with directives or requesting specific things they require done in their environment. GDC are activation of specific mental schemas in the brain from triggers in the external environment. As long as those triggers remain constant in the milieu, GDC persist. (Refer to article on "behaviors based in theories of information processing" for detailed information of this construct).

- If the "busy" states involves activities: such patients are all over the home or the unit, attempting to perform or accomplish activities. From the patient's perspective, each of these activities represents fulfilment of a goal arising from identification of a need from within the patient's immediate environment. GDA are functional in nature. GDA are different from "stimulus bound behaviors" (SBB) and "stereotypical behaviors" (SB). An example of SBB is "utilization behaviors" which are often grasping or groping in nature. Whereas, SB are repetitive, non-functional in nature (see below for examples).

- It is this cohort of behaviors at home or on the unit, which requires the CG or CP to be "chasing after the patients" to prevent them from getting into risk situations. These behaviors create a very high energy milieu and an ongoing challenge for staff to keep patient's safe.

- It is imperative for CG and CP to understand the relationship amongst the "need" for belongingness, motivational drives and fulfilment or satiation of the "need". Patients who exhibit this cohort of behaviors have higher than normal levels of motivational drives due to their dementia/NCD. Fulfilment of the triggered "need" is a necessity for the release of "needs". This is the only way a patient will de-escalate in these circumstances.

- Hence, any responses or interactions by CG or CP which are perceived by the patient as a contradiction or impedance to needs fulfilment will cause a state of increased emotional turmoil. A state of emotional turmoil is congruent with hyper-autonomic arousal which will further increase motivational drives for need fulfilment. The very behaviors being prevented from occurring will escalate further.
- Hence, CG and CP should develop behavioral interventions with a view to providing alternative direction to patient's motivational goals. This would involve creating alternative, more adaptive, activities and not simply attempting to prevent patients from what they are attempting to be doing. As an example, telling the patient who is expressing a thought to go home that he cannot go home will cause emotional distress, thereby increasing motivational drives, thus propelling them further with the desire to go home. Likewise, a patient attempting to rearrange furniture should not be stopped from doing so. Instead, they should be directed to another, similar activity, such as, "can you help me look for your wallet in your room?" or "could you help me fold this laundry first?". Both of these adaptive activities have diverted the high level of energy towards less risky activities thereby successfully diminishing risks associated with initial behaviors.

Specification of the Construct of the Domain

The principle dysregulation underlying the genesis of these behaviors is a varying degree of increase in motivational drives. Merriam-Webster Medical Dictionary (2013) defines "goal-directed" as "aimed toward a goal or towards completion of a task". Goal Directed behaviors can be broken down into two sub-components: goal directed cognitions and goal directed activities.

Goal Directed Cognitions (GDC)

This concept has been described in details in the above section. One of the symptoms of apathy is the absence of goal directed cognition. The absence of GDC is due to a decrease in motivational level in the organism. By reverse, varying degrees of increase in motivational drives will result in a heightened level of interest in interacting with the environment with a subsequent increase ability to recognize the deficiency between the individual's internal state and their environment. Increase in identification of deficiencies will trigger the usual cascade of events identified in the introduction section.

The type of mental schemas activated is determined by the sensory input from the patient's immediate environment. Likewise, the content of the cognitions generated are a direct result of and contingent upon the mental schema activated by the sensory input from the environment. As long as the environment (milieu structure) remains relatively stable over time, content of cognitions remains consistent over those timelines. The following is an example to illustrate this construct.

A patient on an inpatient unit had to move rooms due to a water leak in their room. The sensory input consisted of a snow on the ground outside, their room with an attached bathroom, burst pipes and the water on the floor. All of that evening, the primary cognition expressed by the patient was an intent to go home to turn on the heating to prevent the water pipes from freezing and bursting. The second cognition expressed all of that evening was to go home and organize all the unpaid hydro bills so they could be paid the next morning. All through that evening the patient went between those two cognitions and no amount of redirect by staff was successful in getting the patient away from fixation on those themes. By next evening, the water leak and related damage had all been fixed. On that evening, the patient still wanted to go home but the reasons were to feed the kids and get them ready for school the next morning. The patient remained fixed on that theme through the evening and no degree of redirect could get her away from that theme. This degree of fixation and persistence of these cognitions differentiates it from the phenomenon of confabulation.

Confabulation, by definition, is attempting to fill in the gap or a void in memory during recall of events with fabrications (Baddeley, Kopelman & Wilson, 2003). The facts created to fill the void have no registration, and therefore, no retention and subsequently recall after that moment in time. As an example, when asked what the patient did earlier in the day, the initial response may be they went shopping with their daughter. When asked the same question a half hour later, he/she may tell you they were busy practicing piano all morning. A few hours later, when asked the same question, the patient may tell you they were busy tidying up the house all morning. The patient has remained in that same environment for all this time. As can be seen, there is no consistency of cognitions verbalized along the defined timelines and with the environment staying constant. Goal directed cognitions demonstrate consistency over a given duration of time and as long as the environment remains unchanged.

CG and CP need to understand these conceptual differences between two sets of symptoms as they have major clinical implication in management of the patients.

Goal Directed Activities (GDA)

Persistence of GDC may, can, or will lead to generation of congruent activities. This is governed by the ideomotor principle and the driving forces are motivational levels (Pezzulo et al., 2008). As the motivational levels increase, as happens in various disease states due to changes in autonomic arousal states, there is increased probability of cognitions turning into actions. As an example, a patient who stays fixated on wanting to go home and is unable too, becomes increasingly distraught and upset in their emotional state. This state of emotional upset results in a higher level of autonomic arousal and congruently higher motivational levels. As a consequence, the patient starts to work the handles on the door all over the unit, including, the main entrance. Continued emotional upset will raise the motivational levels even more and this can result in exit-seeking activity or related activities which will aid in exit-seeking. Pulling of the fire alarm may be one such related activity as it will result in opening of the locked door on the unit. It is of paramount to recognize that all the goal directed activities are "functional" in nature. There is a purpose and a meaning to these activities for the patient. They are labeled as "functional motor activities" (FMA). Examples of FMA in dementia/NCD population observed in daily clinical practice are as follows.

Patients with dementia/NCD who have a health care background will invariably start acting as if they work in that environment. They are seen to be transporting patients in wheel chairs to different parts of the ward, strip linen of the beds, an attempt to feed patients or remove them from their beds with a view to transferring them. An attempt to prevent these patients from engaging in such activities creates varying degrees of emotional distress. This results in increased motivational drive and stronger conviction to do even more in the environment. Such patients require redirect with simulated activities which are not associated with the degree of risks associated with activities identified above.

Grandmothers who have lived their lives as home maker will be seen to be moving cutlery and utensils, move linen carts, an attempt to feed patients in wheel chairs which are mistaken as kids in strollers (misidentification behavior). Such patients require engagement in milieu activities like folding linen, setting up or tidying the dining room and dusting the unit as a diversion. It is a common practice to see female patients on dementia/NCD units walking around with dolls and spending all their time caring for them.

Dementia/NCD in patients with various trade backgrounds such as plumbers, carpet layers, electricians will be seen to carrying out related activities on the unit. Using child proof tool boxes and related structures activities on the unit is the most constructive way to engage them instead of preventing them.

In most other scenarios the relationship between patient's background and the observed activities may not be as apparent. Examples of these include rearranging or moving furniture, emptying drawers with a view to packing and then unpacking clothes and pulling down curtains or blinds and plugging the toilets in an attempt to clean them. It is functional nature of these motor activities which differentiate them from "stereotypical" behaviors. The latter are internally driven, non-functional and purposeless activities. The examples of this include rubbing your forehead, taking a cloth to wipe the brow when there is no evidence of its need, or repeatedly touching the door handles while standing in front of the door but there is no effort to pull the door open.

Yet another set of behaviors which need differentiating from goal directed activities are the "stimulus bound" behaviors. By definition, these behaviors are specifically tied to an overt or an obvious stimulus and persist as long as the stimulus persists. Once the stimulus is removed, the behavior ceases to exist. An example of "stimulus bound" behavior is "utilization behavior".

A clinical example of "utilization behaviors" is as follows. A patient, upon seeing a cup, will pick up a spoon and start stirring and will continue to do so as long as the cup remains in sight. Once the cup is removed, the patient may have no use for the spoon. A patient, upon seeing a ball, reaches to pick it up despite being reminded repeatedly to stay in their place. An examiner puts out his hand while simultaneously giving instructions to the patient not to shake his hand. The patient will shake the examiner's hand anyway. These behaviors tend to be more grasping or groping in nature and are directed towards an overt stimulus.

Motor Behaviors

Items in this Category Include:

- Roaming, strolling wandering
- Fidgety, rocking in wheelchair, restless, agitated;
- Seemingly driven, "on the go", wheelchair propelling, chair/bed exiting

Purpose of the Measure or "Meaning of the Behavior"

- Recognition of behaviors in this category is to alert CG and CP of a state of "unrest" in a patient.
- These behaviors, by themselves, do not provide any clues to the reasons for the unrest. They are the most commonly occurring behaviors and garner the most attention in clinical situations. These behaviors make the most background noise in any given clinical situation.
- CG and CP should make an effort to identify the presence of any of the other behavioral categories occurring in conjunction with MB. Only then can an understanding of these behaviors be achieved.

Specification of the Construct of the Category

In literature, motor behaviors have also been labeled as "Wandering Behavior" (WB) (Yokoi et al., 2012). However, in clinical practice, this behavior is routinely labeled as "agitation." WB has been identified as the most commonly occurring and researched behaviors in dementia/NCD (Algase et al., 2010). WB may be classified into two general sub-types: purposeful WB and purposeless WB.

The purposeful wandering, in the present classification system, was included in goal directed behaviors (Yokoi et al., 2012). This behavioral category defines the purposeless WB. "Motor Behaviors" (MB) are the most non-specific symptoms occurring in patients with dementia/NCD. Whether a patient with cognitive impairment is experiencing a major mood, anxiety or psychotic spectrum disorder, an organic mental disorder such as delirium, medication side-effects in the form of akathisia or even a non-pathological state such as an adjustment to a new environment, MB are ubiquitous to each of these presentations. In themselves MB do not help distinguish amongst any of the above fore-mentioned clinical states nor help diagnose any of the above clinical states either. A more beneficial way to conceptualize MB is on the basis of the constructs which define them.

The principal dysregulation in the genesis of this behavioral category is the varying degrees of changes in frequency and amplitude of motor activity. The sum of these two determines the speed of motor activity. The rules of inertia are also applicable to loco-motor disposition and motivational levels are the driving force for loco-motor propulsion with resultant changes in frequency and amplitude of motor activity. The changes in levels of motivation are influenced by the degree of autonomic arousal in the brain and can be the result of a non-pathological state (an adjustment to a new environment) or the sequelae of a disease state (e.g., mood, anxiety or psychotic spectrum disorders, organic mental state as well as delirium).

A decrease in motivation due to lethargy in arousal, as a result of various disease states or medication side-effects, will result in a decrease in speed of motor activity. This results in hypoactive states. Such states are reviewed under "Apathy Behaviors."

Alternatively, an increase in motivational levels will result in an increase in speed of motor activity. As an example, for ambulatory patients, the clinical presentation of roaming, strolling or wandering is due to a minimal increase in arousal with congruent change in frequency and amplitude of motor activity. As the level of arousal increases to moderate levels the frequency and amplitude of motor activity will increase and this could result in emergence of fidgetiness, restlessness and agitation including bed exiting. Further increases in arousal will result in "seemingly driven" and "on the go" type of clinical presentation. Behaviors of being "seemingly driven" or "on the go" should be assessed very carefully to determine if they are antecedents or concomitants to functional motor activities (FMA). If so, they will be captured under GDB.

For patients in wheel chairs, a minimal increase in level of arousal will produce fidgetiness and restlessness in the chair. A moderate increase in arousal can create a state of not being able to sit still including rocking states. As the level of arousal increases further, it may result in wheel chair propelling and chair exiting. Behaviors of being "wheel chair propelling" or "chair exiting" should be assessed very carefully to determine if they antecedents or concomitants to FMA. If so, they will be categorized under GDB.

The milieu further directly shapes how the changes in motor activity, as a consequence of changes in arousal, are labeled. The same degree of motivational change, in two different environments, could be labeled very differently. As an example, a mild degree of increase in motivational level in a smaller crowded environment could be labeled as "restlessness, fidgetiness or agitation" in comparison to a similar increase in a large and an empty environment. In the latter set of circumstances it could be labeled as mere "roaming, strolling or wandering".

Hence, it is reasonable to extrapolate from the above discussions that MB are the most non-specific of all the behaviors in dementia/NCD and are "state" dependent in nature. They do not stay constant and are influenced by the "state of mind" or the "degree of arousal" of the patient. Further, labeling of these behaviors tends to be biased based upon the size of the environment. Hence, it is reasonable to substitute terms like "agitation" and "wandering" with MB as they accurately reflect the concepts underlying these behaviors.

Importuning Behaviors

Items in the Category Include:

- Persistently seeking reassurance or asking for assistance;
- Behaving in ways for demands to be met immediately;
- Shadowing staff; and

- Attention seeking or manipulative behaviors.

Purpose of the Measure or "Meaning of the Behavior"

- Oxford dictionary (2009) defines importuning as "making persistent, insistent or pressing requests to fulfil a need". In context on this behavioral classification, importuning is being used to fulfil physiological needs.
- These are the most innate of human needs and are inclusive of those that are "physical, medical or emotional" in nature. Examples of these include hunger and thirst, need to void or defecate, fatigue and need to rest or sleep, pain or discomfort and seek relief and the need for mental or social stimulation.
- Expression of these needs can be overt or occult and /or obvious or ambiguous.
- Recognition of behaviors in this category is to alert CG and CP to any of the above permutation or combination in the ways in which a "physiological need" may be expressed.
- In the early stages of cognitive impairment, the needs may be expressed via verbal means being overt and obvious. With the progression of cognitive impairment, the expression of these needs becomes more non-verbal, occult and/or ambiguous.
- In the advanced stages of the disease, expression of these needs is likely to take the form of behaviors which are commonly labelled as attention seeking or manipulative. Such expressions are likely to be construed by CG and CP in a negative light thereby potentially resulting in further ignoring of these expressed behaviors. Hence, it may take the form of expression of behaviors which may indeed be counter-productive to the very purpose for which they are being exhibited. Such an interactional dynamic will invariably result in escalation of the behaviors.
- Therefore, behavioral care planning needs to be focused on the identification of these physiological needs in context of these behaviors.

Specification of the Construct of the Category

In review of the literature, "importuning" behaviors have been described in various different clinical situations; sexual deviant behaviors (SDB), addictions behavior (AB), in patients with chronic medical illness, depression and dementia/NCDs.

The most frequent utilization of this term is in context of "soliciting for immoral purposes" in SDB. It is for the purposes of soliciting sex in all different settings. The "need" in these situations is obvious and expressed accordingly. The same principles apply to patient population with addictions. They will seek out emergency rooms, walk-in clinics, and multiple doctors to fulfill that "need" for abuse of prescription medications. Chronic pain is the presenting symptom in all of these situations and these patients can be "persistent, insistent and pressing in request of" their need for medications. The utilization of the term "importuning" in context of patients with chronic medical illness is a bit more heterogeneous. It has been used in context of patients seeking approval for disability pensions from their insurance companies. These patients will present to their health care providers, in a persistent and pressing way, with the same or constantly changing medical signs and symptoms. In patients with hypochondriac disorders, there is a relentless and persistent need to seek medical attention for the fear of having a serious disease. These patients will request extensive investigations in an effort to sooth the fear around having a serious disease. In these situations the "need" is, yet again, obvious.

The use of the term "importuning" in patients with depression has only been used in the elderly population (Lawlor, 1995). The use of "importuning" in dementia/NCD literature has also been in context of "pacing and agitation" (Lawlor, 1995). Literature interprets these behaviors in this patient population as a non-verbal expression of a need which is more ambiguous than obvious. The patient's inability to identify specific needs presents itself in the form of non-specific behaviors. Here again the premise is a non-verbal expression of an ambiguous need although no clear description could be found in the literature. Another context in which importuning has been used in dementia/NCD literature is with "disinhibited behaviors" (Rockwood & MacKnight, 2001). In this context it may be reasonable to extrapolate the use of this term in conjunction with sexually disinhibited behaviors. Of course, the need in these situations will be the same as in SDB though the element of immorality will not be applicable as cognitive impairment will result in loss of self-awareness and self-monitoring (Clare, 2003) in addition to loss of impulse control.

As is evident from above examples, the need may be obvious or ambiguous. Furthermore, the need may be expressed overtly or through non-specific behaviors. Early stages of cognitive impairment may be associated with obvious and overt expression of needs. As the impairment progresses the expression of needs becomes ambiguous and an inability to express it overtly. Hence, behavioral symptoms in the form of persistently seeking staff for reassurance, persistently asking staff for assistance and behavioral manifestations of need for immediate gratification are examples of obvious and overt needs. As the patient progresses through moderate to advanced stages of dementia/NCD, verbal abilities may decline and the patient will express themselves increasingly through nonverbal means. The loss of verbal ability to express their need may be substituted by the patient following the staff all over the ward like their shadow as a way of expressing their need (shadowing of staff). Alternatively, the patients may behave in ways which would draw staffs attention to them with a hope that staff would identify their need (attention seeking). If simple attention seeking does not yield desired results the patients may up the ante and such behaviors may potentially be labeled by staff as manipulative in nature. Behaviors based in importuning can also manifest as "vocal" behaviors in, both, mobile and immobile patients. Examples of this can include calling for a family member, nurse or parents incessantly.

Conclusions

Motivational drives are sub served by preserved motivational circuits in the brain. Motivational drives help in satiation of identified needs. Cognitive impairment due to any etiology may cause disruption in these circuits at varying stages of the disease. Subsequent changes in motivational circuits will impact on drives and congruently impact on either a decrease or an increase in motivational drives.

Apathy behaviors are the result of a decrease in the motivational drives with an absence of any need fulfillment. Goal directed behaviors are the result of an increase in motivational drives with increase in detection and fulfillment of "belongingness" needs. Motor behaviors are the result of varying degrees of changes in motivational drives and occur in conjunction with other identified behavioral categories. Importuning behaviors are the result of preserved motivational drives in detection and fulfillment of physiological needs.

References

Algase, D. L. et al. (1996). Need-driven dementia-compromised behavior: An alternative view of disruptive behavior. *American Journal of Alzheimer's Disease*, 11, 10-19.

Algase, D. L., Beattie, E. R., Antonakos, C., Beel-Bates, C. A., & Yao, L. (2010). Wandering and the physical environment. *American Journal of Alzheimer's Disease and Other Dementias*, 25, 340-346. doi: 10.1177/1533317510365342.

Anderson, R. C. (1977). The Notion of Schemata and the Educational Enterprise: General Discussion of the Conference. In R. C. Anderson, R. J. Spiro, & W. E. Montague (Eds.), *Schooling and the Acquisition of Knowledge.* (pp. 415-431). New Jersey: Lawrence Erlbaum.

Baddeley, A. D., Kopelman, M. D., & Wilson, B. A. (2003). The Cognitive Neuroscience of Cofabulation: A Review and a Model. In A. Gilboa, & M. Moscovitch (Eds.), *The handbook of memory disorders.* (pp. 315 – 342) West Sussex: Wiley.

Clare, L. (2003). Managing threats to self: awareness in early stage Alzheimer's disease. *Social Science & Medicine*, 57, 1017-29. doi: 10.1016/S0277-9536(02)00476-8.

Clarke, D. E., et al. (2008). Apathy in Dementia: Clinical and Sociodemographic Correlates. *The Journal of Neuropsychiatry and Clinical Neurosciences*, 20, 337-347. doi: 10.1176/appi.neuropsych.20.3.337.

Custers, R., & Aarts, H. (2010). The unconscious will: how the pursuit of goals operates outside of conscious awareness. *Science*, 329, 47-50. doi: 10.1126/science.1188595.

Davis, L.L., Buckwalter, K. & Burgio, L.D. (1997). Measuring problem behaviors in dementia: Developing a methodological agenda. *Advances in Nursing Science*, 20, 40-55.

Deci, E. L., & Ryan, R. M. (2000). The "what" and "why" of goal pursuits: Human needs and the self-determination of behavior. *Psychological Inquiry*, 11, 227-268. doi: 10.1207/S15327965PLI1104_01.

Gibson, J. J. (1997). Theory of Affordances. In R. Shaw, & J. Bransford (Eds.), *Perceiving, Acting, and Knowing: Toward an Ecological Psychology.* (pp. 67-82). Hillsdale: Lawrence Erlbaum.

Goal-directed. (2013). In Meriam-Webster Dictionary. Available from: http://www.merriam-webster.com/medical/goal-directed.

Greenwood, P. M. (2007). Functional plasticity in cognitive aging: review and hypothesis. *Neuropsychology*, 21, 657-73. doi: 10.1037/0894-4105.21.6.657.

Hancock, G. A., Woods, B., Challis, D., & Orrell, M. (2006). The needs of older people with dementia in residential care. *International Journal of Geriatric Psychiatry*, 21, 43-49. doi: 10.1002/gps.1421.

Herzberg, F., Mausner, B., & Snyderman, B. B. (1959). *The Motivation to Work.* New York: John Wiley.

Importune. (2010). In Oxford Dictionaries. Available from: http://oxforddictionaries.com/definition/english/importune?q=importuni ng

Kovach, C. R., Noonan, P. E., Schlidt, A. M., & Wells, T. (2005). A model of consequences of need-driven, dementia-vompromised behavior. *Journal of Nursing Scholarship*, 37, 134-140.
doi: 10.1111/j.1547-5069.2005.00025_1.x.

Landes, A. M., Sperry, S. D., Strauss, M. E., & Geldmacher, D. S. (2001). Apathy in Alzheimer's disease. *Journal of the American Geriatrics Society*, 49, 1700-7. doi: 10.1046/j.1532-5415.2001.49282.x.

Lawlor, B. A. (Ed.). (1995). *Behavioral complications in Alzheimer's disease* (pp. 31). Washington: American Psychiatric Press.

Locke, E. A., Shaw, K. N., Saari, L. M., & Latham, G. P. (1981). Goal setting and task performance: 1969-1980. *Psychological Bulletin*, 90, 125-152. doi: 10.1037/0033-2909.90.1.125.

Luthra, A.S. (2013). *Classification of behaviors in dementia based in impairment in theories based upon information processing pathways.* Manuscript submitted for publication.

Marin, R. S., & Wilkosz, P. A. (2005). Disorders of diminished motivation. *Journal of Head Trauma Rehabilitation*, 20, 377-88.
doi: 10.1097/00001199-200507000-00009.

Maslow, A. H. (1943). A theory of human motivation. *Psychological Review*, 50, 370-96. doi: 10.1037/h0054346.

McClelland, D. C. (1967). *The Achieving Society.* New York: Free Press.

Mega, M. S., Cummings, J. L., Fiorello, T., & Gornbein, J. (1996). The spectrum of behavioral changes in Alzheimer's disease. *Neurology*, 46, 130-135. doi: 10.1212/WNL.46.1.130.

Pezzulo, G., Butz, M. V., Castelfranchi, C., & Falcone, R. (2008). *The challenge of anticipation: A unifying framework for the analysis and design of artificial cognitive systems* (Eds.). Germany: Springer.

Rockwood, K. & MacKnight, C. (2001). Behaviour Disturbances. In *Understanding dementia: a primer of diagnosis and management.* (pp. pp 163-166, 167, 171, 177) Halifax, NS: Pottersfield Press.

Skinner, B. F. (1953). *Science and human behavior.* New York: Macmillan.

Starkstein, S. E., & Leentjens, A. F. (2008). The nosological position of apathy in clincial practice. *Journal of Neurology, Neurosurgery & Psychaitry*, 79, 1088-1092. doi: jnnp.2007.136895v1.

Vroom, V. H. (1964). *Work and motivation.* New York: Wiley.

Yokoi, T., Aoyama, K., Ishida, K., & Okamura, H. (2012). Conditions Associated With Wandering in People With Dementia From the Viewpoint of Self-

Awareness Five Case Reports. *American Journal of Alzheimer's Disease and Other Dementias*, 27, 162-170. doi: 10.1177/1533317512442995.

Chapter 6: Classification of Behaviors in Dementia/NCDs based upon Theories of Regulation of Emotion

This chapter is focused on the third theoretical construct of behaviors based upon "theories on regulation of emotions". Behavioral categories emanating from "theories on regulation of emotions" are the result of impairment in the neuronal structures and circuits in the brain which are involved in the generation and regulation of emotions. This impairment in regulation of emotions is a direct consequence of cognitive impairment; irrespective of the etiology. In order to understand the implications of the impairment of emotional circuits on generation of behaviors, it is imperative to understand the structure and function of these circuits in individuals with normal cognitive function.

Concept of Emotions and Moods

The terms "emotions" and "moods" are distinct and separate, requiring an independent understanding. Both have significant clinical implications in the context of dementia/NCD.

Parkinson et al. (1996) and Clore, Schwarz and Conway (1994) have provided many of the distinguishing features between "emotions" and "moods". According to Parkinson et al. (1996), emotions have the following characteristics:

i.   Emotions always arise in context of a specific situation. These situations can be extrinsic (environment) or intrinsic (mental representations)

ii.   Emotions are experienced as a "whole body phenomenon." Emotional components include subjective experience, behavioral, central, and peripheral physiological changes (Mauss et al., 2005). These were initially classified as "experiential", "behavioral" and "physiological" responses, respectively. The subjective experience is the "feeling state" and the term emotions is used synonymously with feelings

iii. Emotions have an imperative quality termed as "control precedence", meaning that emotions can force their way into our awareness thereby interrupting whatever we are doing (Frijda, 1986)

iv.   Emotional responses lead to a dynamic process by often modifying or changing the situation which initially gave rise to these emotions

According to Clore, Schwarz and Conway (1994), moods have the following characteristics:

i.   Moods tend to be persistent, last much longer, and are not situation specific
ii.   Moods are more diffuse and more tied to cognitions than actions;
iii.   Moods lack "control precedence" and
iv.   Moods do not always modify or change situations.

Limitations in Assessment of Mood in Moderate to Advanced Dementia/NCD

When the subjective recall is relatively preserved, as is the case in Mild Cognitive Impairment, or in the very early stages of dementia/NCD, it is reasonable to elucidate changes in mood with some degree of accuracy and work within the established DSM parameters. However, it is vitally important to make the distinction between emotions and mood in patients with moderate to advanced stages of dementia/NCD. Advancing cognitive impairment is likely to make subjective recall of "mood" rather unreliable due to failing memory and self-awareness. The reliability and validity of a response to a question such as; "how would you rate your mood over the last 2 weeks?" or "has there been a decline in your interest levels or pleasure" in a patient with moderate to advanced stages of dementia/NCD must be challenged. The wording alone is abstract as is the construct and in excess of this patients ability to accurately grasp and subsequently report on it. This, in turn, would challenge the reliability and validity of a diagnosis of a Major Depressive Episode in patients with moderate to advanced dementia/NCD.

Standardized scales are utilized used in dementia/NCD care to rate the severity of depression. Examples include *Cornell Scale for Depression in Dementia/NCD* (CSDD) (Alexopoulos et al., 1988) and *Dementia/NCD Mood Assessment Scale* (Sunderland et al., 1988). However, the primary role of these scales reiterated is to measure the severity of depression and not to be used as a screening or a diagnostic tool in this cohort (Visser et al., 2000). Unfortunately, utilization as a diagnostic tool is a common misuse of these scales in clinical practice. Yet, Alexopoulos et al. (1988) in their original article emphasized, "The Cornell scale is a quantitative measure of depression. Although, its total scores correlate with the presence of depressive syndromes classified by RDC, the Cornell scale is not designed for the use as a diagnostic instrument".

A comparable analogy would be to use Braden's scale for staging the severity of pressure sores when its primary role is to predict the risk of occurrence of pressure sores (Bergstrom et al., 1987). It is simply not intended for this use. It cannot and should not be utilized for anything alternatively than its intended; an all too common a practice with CSDD. It is extremely unreliable to establish persistence of dysregulation in moods and or interest and pleasure over longer (2 weeks) duration of time. So, because they cannot self-report on mood and we lack valid and reliable scale for diagnosing, it is being proposed we monitor changes in emotional responses in patients with moderate to advanced stages of dementia/NCD.

Reasons to Assess Emotions in Moderate to Advanced Dementia/NCD

Another very important concept in understanding of emotional symptoms was placed forth by Shimokawa, et al. (2001). They studied the concept of emotional comprehension, its association with cognitive impairment, and its role in interpersonal behaviors. Shimokawa, et al. (2001) proved that decline in cognitive abilities is not congruent with a decline in emotional comprehension. Emotional comprehension tends to be preserved for longer well into the advanced stages of cognitive impairment.

There is evidence that older adults are more emotionally expressive than younger adults (Malatesta-Magai et al., 1992). Further evidence supports that emotional expressivity is not only preserved, even heightened in older patients with cognitive impairment (Lang & Carstensen, 1994). Lawton, et al. (1996) established that all streams of emotions, such as anger, joy, melancholy and fear, continue to be expressed in patients with cognitive impairment. Magai et al. (1996) further elucidated the expression of joy and pleasure are diminished in late stages of cognitive impairment, but those of anger, fear, and melancholy are well preserved to heightened in similar circumstances.

Emotions in all human beings are expressed in two forms: non-verbally, performed physically through facial, vocal and postural displays; and verbally, through communicated language. The expression of emotions is regulated through two processes: intrinsic processes, including acquired or learned strategies of self-management; and extrinsic, including social partners, life circumstances, milieu structure and mood regulating agents. There are five factors which influence this emotional regulatory process (Gross, 1998):

    i.   Situation selection
    ii.   Situation modification
    iii.   Attention deployment
    iv.   Cognitive schema change or reframing
    v.   Response modulation

Situation selection and *modification* refer to the individual's ability to change the environment or contents within the environment to influence emotions. *Attention deployment* refers to an individual's ability to use diversion or distractions methods to diminish the impact of the situation thereby decreasing the emotional response. *Cognitive reframing* refers to an individual's ability to assimilate the situation into their mental schema and restructure the schema, thereby decreasing the emotional response. These first four factors require the patient to have a relative degree of intellectual preservation in order to modify the generation of emotions. Unfortunately, with failing intellectual abilities, as is the case in moderate to advanced dementia/NCD, patients become incapable of modifying any of these four variables on their own and require care givers (CG) or care providers (CP) to take charge of the situation to modify emotions. The last factor involved in regulating emotions is *response modulation*. Most of the response modulation is attained with a combined approach of use of medications along with interpersonal and environmental interventions from CG or CP.

Generation and regulation of emotions occur simultaneously. There is a bidirectional link between the limbic system, which generates emotions, and cortical centers, which regulate emotion (Gross, 2009). Advancing stages of dementia/NCD impair the neuronal circuits in the limbic and cortical systems thereby impairing or compromising the stimulus appropriate generation and regulation of emotions in this patient population. The dysregulation in the proportional generation of emotions in addition to patients diminished ability to regulate factors which influence emotions results in a perpetual state of emotional instability.

Classification of Emotions

Plutchik (1980) has classified emotions into primary and secondary emotions. There are five main primary emotions experienced by human beings:

    i.   Sadness or melancholy
   ii.   Discontentment
  iii.   Fear
  iv.   Anger
   v.   Joy or Happiness

Primary emotions combine to generate secondary emotions. Examples of secondary emotions include optimism, love, awe, disappointment, remorse, contempt and aggression. The purpose of this article is to categorize emotional behaviors in dementia/NCD using the suggested classifications. Discontentment is the only primary emotion which seems to coexist with, both, melancholy and anger (Plutchik ,1980). Classifications of behaviors based upon principles of emotional regulation include the following:

    I.   Emotional Behaviors (EB), encompassing verbal and non-verbal behaviors expressed through emotions of melancholy and discontentment
   II.   Fretful/Trepidated Behaviors (FTB), encompassing verbal and non-verbal behaviors expressed through emotions of fear;
  III.   Vocal Behaviors (VB); aggressive and effusive type, encompassing verbal and non-verbal behaviors expressed through emotions of anger and discontentment (vocal behaviors; aggressive type) and emotions of joy (vocal behaviors; effusive type)

Melancholy, Discontentment, and Fear

Emotions of melancholy and fear are viewed as negative in nature having several other similarities. Expressions of melancholy and fear, in any given environment, are governed by four principles:

1. Maximization of positive effect
2. Minimization of negative effect
3. Minimization of affective inhibition
4. Means-ends competence to achieve above three principles (Gross, 2009)

Emotional regulation involves monitoring, evaluating, and adjusting affective responses to changes in the environment (Gross, 2009). Hence, the principles which govern the expression of these emotions and the processes that regulate these emotions serve the purpose of catharsis in a measured way and to allow for decompression from pain or pain experience (Gross, 2009). Even though from an observer's perspective, these emotions may represent suffering, from a patient's perspective all of these behaviors are comforting.

In essence, the above four principles translate into an organism placing forth efforts to allow themselves to feel good all the time, diminish exposure to pain and distress, and be able to express all of these emotions without limitations or barriers.

Criteria and format put forth by Davis, Buckwalter and Burgio (1997) will be used structure the behavioral category. According to Davis, Buckwalter and Burgio (1997), the criteria to describe behaviors are as follows: identification of the target population, specification of the "construct" of the category or domain, purpose of the measure, and items in behavioral category. This criteria and format was chosen due to its relevancy to classifying behavioral symptoms in dementia/NCD and its widespread acceptability, as it is commonly cited and used in research regarding behavior in persons with dementia/NCD or related mental health disorders; and its application to behavioral management of dementia/NCD and related mental health disorders in acute and long term care settings.

Emotional Behaviors

Items in the Emotional Behavior Category Include:

*   Appearing sad, despondent or tearful
*   Expression of despair, morbidity, gloominess and helplessness;
*   Mimicking or mocking and being dismissive
*   Sarcastic or Teasing, derogatory comments, being critical and negative of others
*   Feeling rejected or increased sensitivity to comments from others

Purpose of the Category or "Meaning of the Behavior"

- Emotions of melancholy and discontentment are viewed to be negative in nature and cause pain. We, as human beings, tend to spend substantial amounts of energy to minimize the impact of this pain in our daily existence. The emotional regulatory mechanism which govern the expression of these emotions and processes which regulate these emotions serve one primary purpose of "catharsis", in a measured way, in order to allow for decompression from pain. While, from an observer's perspective these emotions represent suffering. From the patient's perspective they are comforting in nature. These behaviors are meant to decrease pain, decrease exposure to risk of being hurt and result in feeling good.

- Expression of these behaviors serves the purpose of soliciting comforting responses from CG and CP. Such responses allow for a measured catharsis of the pain. All care planning around non-verbal and verbal behaviors of melancholy should focus on enhancing a safe and a structured environment in which these behaviors can be expressed.

- Verbal and non-verbal expressions discontentment serve the purpose of preventing exposure to the risk of being hurt resulting in pain.

- Making derogatory comments, being sarcastic or negative of others, mimicking or mocking others serves two purposes for the patient. First is to feel good about oneself by putting other people down. Secondly, HSP (individuals who are "thin skinned"), it serves the purpose of shutting down all lines of communication with others thereby preventing any hurt or pain in future interactions. These behaviors help patients reject others before they can be rejected, an experience associated with pain and hurt.

- These dynamics also apply to the patients interactions with CG and CP. These behaviors risk being judged by CG and CP as "arrogant". Such labelling results in CG and CP actively avoiding or rejecting the patient. This perceived avoidance or rejection by CG and CP causes emotional pain; paradoxically the very experience patients want to avoid in interactions with others. This will escalate the index behavior. CG and CP need to recognize the underlying dynamics and, at all times, should remain embracing and accepting in their demeanour with the patients. Consistency in exhibition of such a demeanour by CG and CP will ultimately allow the patient to feel accepted and put aside the notion of rejection and pain, despite their maladaptive approach to that very end.

Specification of the Construct of the Category

Emotional behaviors reflect a constellation of sign and symptoms based in melancholy and discontentment. In a clinical setting, it is relatively easy to pick out non-verbal and verbal expressions of melancholy and discontentment. The key to detecting non-verbal and verbal expressions is to carefully listen to and observe patients in their milieu. Non-verbal expression of melancholy takes the form of appearing sad, despondent, or tearful. Verbal expressions of melancholy are based in themes of despair, morbidity, gloominess, and pervasive hopelessness. Non-verbal expressions of discontentment take the form of mimicking or mocking behaviors, being dismissive of others, and having a sarcastic disposition. Verbal expressions of discontentment take the form of teasing others or making derogatory comments, being critical of and possessing a pervasive sense of negativity towards everything and everyone, feeling rejected, or increased sensitivity to comments made by others.

As stated earlier, the purpose in expression of non-verbal and verbal communication for the organism is to feel good, decrease pain and hurt or the risk of being hurt. This goal is achieved in the following manner for all the symptoms identified:

- Expressing sadness or tearfulness. These themes of morbidity and despair allow for safe decompression and catharsis of painful emotions and assists in seeking comfort from others. CG and CP respond accordingly to provide solace to the patient thereby decreasing pain
- Making derogatory comments, being critical of others, or negativity directed towards others are viewed by recipients as "put-downs". Although communicating in this way helps the patients feel more content within themselves and better about themselves, in comparison to others. This process is automatic and outside the conscious awareness in patients with moderate to advanced dementia/NCD. This approach helps individuals elevate their own self-worth by devaluing others
- Interpersonal interactions between or amongst individuals can be either pleasant or unpleasant. Individuals characterized as *highly sensitive persons* (HSP) tend to be extremely sensitive to comments made by others (Aron, 1997). They more vulnerable, in comparison to healthy individuals, to being emotionally hurt (the opposite of "thick-skinned"). Hence, nonverbal expression of mimicking, mocking and being dismissive and verbal expressions of being sarcastic or teasing tends to shut down all lines of communication with individuals in the milieu. Such an expression provides a protective defense mechanism for individuals in order to reduce exposure to hurt and pain. In a way these individuals, in a proactive manner, compensate for the fear of rejection by others by rejecting them first.

Fretful/Trepidation Behaviors

Items in the Fretful/Trepidation Behavior Category Include:

- Fearful or scared facial expressions
- Anxious or distressed facial expressions
- Clingy or "latches on", ringing of hands, rubbing face or body
- Expressing worry, fear, foreboding or catastrophe

Purpose of the Category or "Meaning of the Behavior"

- Recognition of the behaviors in this category is to make CG and CP aware of the profound sense of 'insecurity' being experienced by the patient in their immediate environment.
- In the hierarchy of human needs, "security needs" follow the fulfilment of "physiological needs". Security needs require the individual to attach to a "secure base" in their environment to feel safe. The attachment to the secure base only occurs if the base is receptive and responsive. The type of attachment formed in the developmental years carries an individual through their life spectrum (secure, avoidant, anxious or disorganized). These attachments are stored as mental schemas in the brain and guide individuals throughout their life spectrum (Nevid, 2012).
- Suffice it to say, these set of behaviors are likely to occur in patients who had mal-adaptive attachment styles (avoidant, anxious or disorganized) through their developmental years.
- Through various stages of cognitive impairment, patients will attempt to pair familiar triggers in their environment with the stored mental schemas. The type of attachments developed will be determined by attachment styles from their developmental years.
- Once all external familiarity fades, as occurs in moderate to advanced stages of dementia/NCD, patients will turn inwards and invoke mental schemas of their loved ones to feel safe. The earliest attachments are to ones parents and hence the concept of parent fixation in advanced stages of dementia/NCDs. Here again, the type of attachments formed will be determined by early developmental styles.
- The goal of non-medical interventions is to identify the secure base from their life and recreate it in the present milieu. Interventions can range from moving old furniture into the new milieu, displaying pictures of immediate family or those from family of origin or work related memorabilia from there past. Hence, the application of reminiscing with recreational therapist, memory book or shadow boxes outside the rooms in long term care facilities.

Specification of the Construct of the Domain

Bowlby (1973) proposed the "attachment theory" as a fundamental basis to forming relationships. The basic underpinnings of this theory were that individuals need relationships, not only for emotional and social development, but also for their preservation. These relationships are only formed with those individuals who are receptive and responsive in nature.

Once these attachments are formed, they result in the development of "internal working models", commonly referred to as mental schemas, which guide individuals through periods of environmental perturbations (Nevid, 2012). Ainsworth (1969) expanded this theory further to introduce the concept of a "secure base". Using the principles of "secure base", Ainsworth and Bell (1970) proposed different types of "attachment models". These were contingent upon the strength of the bond to the "secure base" and included: secure, avoidant, anxious, and disorganized attachments.

The key to developing any of the above types of attachments is the manner in which the individuals, to which the attachments are being formed, respond to such approaches. The initial research was conducted with infants and toddlers. The individuals or secure base in question were the mothers. Literature further supports the applicability of these same principles in the development of peer relationships of all ages, inclusive of romantic relationships, relationships during times of illness or stress and in the elderly (Ainsworth, 1989).

Antonucci (1994) validated the "attachment theory" in older adults. Miesen (1992) elaborated further researching the relationship between advanced stages of cognitive impairment and "attachment theory" in patients with dementia/NCDs. Based on his results he coined the term "parent fixation". According to this term, many patients with dementia/NCDs continue to hold a belief that one or both of their parents are still alive and invoke their memories as a way of creating a secure base.

In the early stages of cognitive impairment patients retain their ability to recognize faces in the environment and the environment itself. Recognition of familiar faces and environment triggers contextual mental schemas of past attachments and generate congruent emotional responses. If the attachment models are secure in nature, subsequent behaviors will be adaptive; however, if the attachment models are anxious or disorganized, subsequent behaviors will be reflective of this and maladaptive for the patient.

As the degree of cognitive impairment advances and the recognition of familiarity of faces and environment fails, patients invoke inner working models of their loved ones to establish security. The purpose of this attempt to connect to inner working models is to diminish themes of uncertainty in their environment and regulate emotions of fear. The loss of memory in dementia/NCD is reciprocal in nature; the information learned last is forgotten first and the information learned first last forgotten. Depending on the severity of the stage of dementia/NCD the patient invokes congruent inner working models. For example, in the moderate stage of dementia/NCD they may invoke inner working models of their relationships to their spouses, friends or children. In the advanced stages of dementia/NCD they may invoke mental schemas of parent fixation as described above. The type of attachment patients have had with their spouses, friends, children, or parents will determine the behavioral presentation in that individual. If the attachment style was secure, the patients will continue to successfully invoke the 'inner working models' to provide them with a secure base. In these patients, they will not display or exhibit any non-verbal or verbal expression of fear or insecurity. If on the other hand, the underlying attachment style was either anxious or disorganized, the patients will invoke inner working models which will not provide them with a secure base. These patients are likely to express this internal insecurity and fear through non-verbal and verbal means. Hence, in the early stages of cognitive impairment, the patients may be able to form attachments with animate and inanimate objects in their environment to feel safe and gain a sense of security (provided their inner working models are secure type). If the inner working models are any of the other two types, anxious or disorganized, FTBs will emerge.

Once again, the emergence of behaviors, or not, will be determined by pre-morbid attachment styles. Non-verbal expressions of these behaviors include: fearful, worried, or scared facial expressions; ringing hands, appearing timid, and rubbing face or body; and appearing clingy and showing a "latch-on" disposition. Verbal expressions include verbalizing fear and worry, foreboding, and themes of catastrophe.

It has been the writer's clinical experience that in immobile patients, due to their inability to seek out comfort in their milieu by physically approaching others, they tend to call out for help (vocal behavior). Hence, the need to recognize one subtype of VB based in fretfulness.

Anger, Discontentment, Joy

Emotions of anger and discontentment and emotions of joy will be addressed in this part of the paper, with focus on vocal behaviors.

Vocal Behaviors

Items in the vocal behavior category include:

- Explosiveness, argumentative and quarrelsome
- Talking loud and fast, acting manic-like
- Whimpering, moaning, making strange noises, yelling and screaming
- Persistent calling out for staff/family or parents
- Rattling bedrails, banging tabletops

Purpose of the Category or "Meaning of the Behavior"

For verbal behavior regarding the aggressive type, recognition of behaviors in this category is to make CG and CP aware of the defensive and attack nature of interactions by the patients in their immediate environment. The purpose of the "defensive" mode, for the patient, is to prevent further exposure to a perceived noxious stimulus in their immediate environment. These behaviors take the form of explosiveness. These behaviors are to be viewed by CG or CP as a "shot across the bow" by the patient. CG or CP should heed to this warning signal and attempt to identify possible triggers in the immediate milieu as being contributory. These triggers will need to be extinguished to prevent further escalation in behaviors. Continued presence of these perceived noxious stimuli runs the risk of pushing the behavior into an "attack" mode. These behaviors may take the form of becoming argumentativeness and quarrelsome. Continued escalation of these behaviors may result in physical aggression directed towards the noxious stimuli. These behaviors should also alert the CG or CP to the "out of proportion'" responses of dementia/NCD patients to various perceived noxious stimuli. When attempting to interact with dementia/NCD patients under these circumstances, CG or CP should make an effort to calibrate their own emotional responses such that patient's behaviors do not get pushed from a "defensive" to an "attack" mode.

Talking fast and loud, acting manic-like: These behavioral symptoms represent the expression of the primary emotion of happiness. These symptoms included under the category of VB effusive type. Recognition of symptoms in this category is to make CG or CP aware of the excitable and "out of proportion" responses of dementia/NCD patients to pleasant stimuli in their environment. CG and CP should make an effort to create a low stimulation environment to diminish the "out of proportion" responses in such circumstances. When attempting to interact with dementia/NCD patients under these circumstances, CG or CP should make an effort to calibrate their own emotional responses such that patient's behaviors do not escalate any further. This is because CG or CP need to remain cognizant of the risks associated with these 'out of proportion" responses to pleasurable stimuli in the environment. Amongst the risks identified are emergence of sexual behaviors or emotional instability leading to verbal and/or physical aggression.

Specification of the Construct of the Category

Dysregulation in emotions of anger with discontentment and emotions of joy have their basis in the principles of emotional vulnerability and individuals' ability to regulate emotional responses and the interaction between the two. Emotional vulnerability is characterized by a marked sensitivity to emotional stimuli (low threshold) and unusually strong reactions (high amplitude) that are abnormally slow in returning to baseline (long duration) (Donegan et al., 2003). Abnormalities in emotional vulnerability result in changes in intensity of expression of these emotions. Emotional instability is a phenomenon of lack of an individual's ability to internally regulate emotions. Cognitive impairment can cause impairment of both emotional vulnerability' and the ability to adequately regulate emotions. The onset of cognitive impairment impacts on emotional vulnerability in a way that the "degree of sensitivity to emotional stimuli" is increased (low threshold), strength of reaction is intensified (high amplitude) and the time to return to baseline is unusually prolonged (longer duration) (Donegan et al., 2003). In addition, there is reduced comprehension capacity of the brain such that even the simplest of the stimuli can be perceived as complex and overwhelming. Consequently, there is increased propensity to being overwhelmed by noxious, non-noxious, and even ambiguous stimuli from within the environment.

    In a clinical setting, this would present itself as an "out of proportion" response to a given stimuli. Such a response in emotions of anger and discontentment are clinically labeled as catastrophic reactions (CR) (Goldstein, 1995). Golstein (1995) defined CR as the, "reaction of the organism when unable to cope with a serious defect in physical and cognitive functions." He described the CR as a short-lasting emotional outburst characterized by anxiety, tears, aggressive behavior, swearing, displacement, refusal, renouncement, and/or compensatory boasting. The CR was further described as inadequate, disordered, inconstant, and inconsistent reactions, embedded in physical and mental shock (Goldstein, 1995). This phenomenon is also referred to as "affective hyper-reactivity" (AH). Similar out of proportion response in emotions of joy will present themselves as manic-like behaviors.

    Yet another manifestation of dysregulation in emotions of anger and discontentment is in the form of dysphoric episodes. Dysphoria is defined as an internally driven feeling of being miserable, crabby, irritable and angry (Starcevic, 2007). The term dysphoria has been used in psychiatric literature in many different contexts, such as:

- Dysphoria episode (DE), representing the irritable-quarrelsome-destructive (IQD) phase of mania of bipolar disorder (BD) (Starcevic, 2007)
- Dysphoria being used interchangeably with depressed mood (Starcevic, 2007);
- Dysphoria being used to define mixed states of BD (Starcevic, 2007)

There is an obvious lack of consensus in use of this term in psychiatric literature (Starcevic, 2007) and it is outside the scope of this article to build consensus on the use of this term. Yet, none of these terms specifically address the phenomenon of dysphoria in relationship to behaviors in dementia/NCD.

For the purposes of discussion in this article, DE will be used to represent the IQD syndrome in patients with dementia/NCD. This syndrome has been described in BD literature in the manic phase of the disease. Factor analysis of different clinical states of BD identifies varied symptom clusters and IQD represents one such cluster. This cluster or syndrome consists of symptoms of profound irritability, anger and discontentment, motor agitation and racing thoughts, loud speech, and associated distrust and suspicion with functional motor activities. These functional motor activities are almost always destructive in nature; either towards oneself or towards objects, property or people in the milieu. With the exception of racing thoughts all other symptoms can be identified on clinical observation. In patients with early stages of dementia/NCD symptoms of racing thoughts can be elicited in a clinical interview. As the dementia/NCD progresses through moderate to advanced stages, it becomes difficult to elicit subjective symptoms of racing thoughts. In such cases, symptoms of distractibility, hyper vigilance and scanning of the environment may be the behavioral manifestations of a racing mind. This cluster of signs and symptoms can escalate to a level of destructiveness in interpersonal interactions (IPI) or towards the environment. When it takes place in the context of IPI it can take the form of a physical attack towards staff. When it is directed towards the environment it presents as destruction of property. When it is directed towards one self, it presents as self-destructive behaviors.

Specific areas in the brain have been identified to be associated with dysregulation in emotions of anger and discontentment (Sander et al., 2005). Such a dysregulation may or may not be associated with an increase in functional motor activity (FMA). When the emotional dysregulation is not associated with FMA it becomes a part of defensive behavior (Vasanthapuram, 2011). When the emotional dysregulation is associated with FMA it becomes a component of "attack" behaviors (Vasanthapuram, 2011). These emotional dysregulation principles are applicable to concepts of AH and DE in patients with moderate to advanced stages of dementia/NCD. AH is a form of catastrophic reaction which is not associated with FMA and should be labeled as a defensive behavior. The primary purpose of this behavior is to prevent further exposure to noxious stimuli within the environment. DE is a form of catastrophic reaction associated with

FMA of destructiveness towards individuals and property within the environment. It should be labeled as an "attack" behavior. Hence, DE is additionally a form of "goal directed activity". The primary purpose of this behavior is to make an attempt to obliterate the noxious stimuli. DE can be viewed as an extension of AH as long as the noxious stimuli persist in the environment.

Conclusions

It is imperative to make distinction between concepts of emotions and moods in context of dementia/NCD patients. Establishing persistence in abnormalities of mood can be extremely challenging in patients with advanced stages of dementia/NCD. Identifying primary emotions and understanding the relationship between cognitive impairment and emotions and their dysregulation in disease states is a preferable approach in these circumstances.

Pathology in expression of primary emotions of melancholy is to provide the patient with a measured catharsis and to allow for decompression from pain. Pathology in expression of primary emotions of discontentment is to protect the patient from pain and hurt. Pathology in expression of emotions of fear is to make CG or CP aware of the profound sense of insecurity being experienced by the patient in a given environment. Pathology in expression of emotions of anger and joy is to highlight the out of proportion nature of responses in these patients. These out of proportion responses may or may not be associated with FMA. If the responses are associated with FMA, they would qualify as goal-directed behaviors. FMA associated with emotion of anger can help understand destructive behaviors in these patients. FMA associated with emotions of joy can help understand "manic-like" behaviors in these patients.

References

Ainsworth, M. D. (1989). Attachments beyond infancy. *American Psychologist*, 44, 709-716. doi: 10.1037/0003-066X.44.4.709.

Ainsworth, M. D. (1969). Object relations, dependency, and attachment: a theoretical review of the infant-mother relationship. *Child Development*, 40, 969-1025.

Ainsworth, M. D., & Bell, S. M. (1970). Attachment, exploration, and separation: illustrated by the behavior of one-year-olds in a strange situation. *Child Development*, 41, 49-67.

Alexopoulos, G. S., Abrams, R. C., Young, R. C., & Shanoian, C. A. (1988). Cornell Scale for depression in dementia. *Biological Psychiatry*, 23, 271-84. doi: 10.1016/0006-3223(88)90038-8.

Antonucci, T. C. (1994). Attachment in adulthood and aging. In M. B. Sperling, & W. H. Berman (Eds.), *Attachment in adults: Clinical and developmental perspectives.* (pp. 256-272). New York: Guilford Press.

Aron, E. N. (1996). The Highly Sensitive Person. New York: Broadway.

Bergstrom, N., Braden, B. J., Laguzza, A., & Holman, V. (1987). The Braden Scale for predicting pressure sore risk. *Nursing Research*, 36, 205-210. doi: 10.1097/00006199-198707000-00002.

Bowlby, J. (1973). *Attachment and loss* (Vol. 2). New York: Basic Books.

Clore, G. L., Schwarz, N., & Conway, M. (1994). Affective causes and consequences of social information processing. In R. S. Wyer Jr., & T. K. Srull (Eds.), *Handbook of social cognition*, 2nd edition. (pp. 323-418). Hillsdale, NJ: Erlbaum.

Davis, L. L., Buckwalter, K., & Burgio, L. D. (1997). Measuring problem behaviors in dementia: developing a methodological agenda. *Advances in Nursing Science*, 20, 40-55.

Donegan, N. H., et al. (2003). Amygdala hyperreactivity in Borderline Personality Disorder: Implications for emotional dysregulation. *Biological Psychiatry*, 54, 1284-1293. doi: 10.1016/S0006-3223(03)00636-X.

Frijda, N. H. (1986). *The emotions*. Cambridge: Cambridge University Press.

Goldstein, K. (1995). *The Organism: A Holistic Approach to Biology Derived from Pathological Data in Man*. New York: Zone Books.

Gross, J. J. (1998). The Emerging Field of Emotion Regulation: An Integrative Review. *Review of General Psychology*, 2, 271-299. doi: 10.1037/1089-2680.2.3.271.

Gross, J. J. (Ed.). (2009). *Handbook of emotion regulation*. New York: The Guilford Press.

Lang, F. R., & Carstensen, L. L. (1994). Close emotional relationships in late life: further support for proactive aging in the social domain. *Psychology and Aging*, 9, 315-324. doi: 10.1037/0882-7974.9.2.315.

Lawton, M. P., Van Haitsma, K., & Klapper, J. (1996). Observed affect in nursing home residents with Alzheimer's disease. *Journals of Gerontology: Series B Psychology Science and Social Science*, 51, 3-14. doi: 10.1093/geronb/51B.1.P3.

Luthra, A.S. (2013). *New Terminology to Label Behaviors in Dementias: Stage Congruent Responsive Behaviors (SCRB)*. Manuscript submitted for publication.

Luthra, A.S. (2013). *Classification of behaviors in dementia/NCD based in impairment in theories based upon information processing pathways*. Manuscript submitted for publication.

Luthra, A.S. (2013). *Classification of Behaviors in DementiaBased in "Motivational" and "Needs Based" Theories*. Manuscript submitted for publication.

Magai, C., Cohen, C., Gomberg, D., Malatesta, C., & Culver, C. (1996). Emotional expression during mid- to late-stage dementia. *International Psychogeriatrics*, 8, 383-395. doi: 10.1017/S104161029600275X.

Malatesta-Magai, C., Jonas, R., Shepard, B., & Culver, L. C. (1992). Type A behavior pattern and emotion expression in younger and older adults. *The Psychology of Aging*, 7, 551-561. doi: 10.1037/0882-7974.7.4.551.

Mauss, I. B., Levenson, R. W., McCarter, L., Wilhelm, F. H., & Gross, J. J. (2005). The tie that binds? Coherence among emotion experience, behavior, and physiology. *Emotion*, 5, 175-190. doi: 10.1037/1528-3542.5.2.175.

Miesen, B. M. (1992). Attachment theory and dementia. In G. M. Jones, & B. M. Miesen (Eds.), *Care-giving in Dementia*. (pp. 38-56). London: Routledge.

Nevid, J.S. (2012). *Psychology: Concepts and Applications Third Edition.* Belmont: Wadsworth Cengage Learning.

Parkinson, B., Totterdell, P., Briner, R. B., & Reynolds, S. (1996). *Changing moods: The psychology of mood and mood regulation.* London: Addison Wesley Longman.

Plutchik, R. (1980). *Emotion, a psychoevolutionary synthesis.* New York: Harper & Row.

Sander, D., Grandjean, D., Pourtois, G., Schwartz, S., Seghier, M. L., Scherer, K. R., & Vuilleumier, P. (2005). Emotion and attention interactions in social cognition: Brain regions involved in processing anger prosody. *Neuroimage, 28,* 848-858. doi: 10.1016/j.neuroimage.2005.06.023.

Shimokawa, A. et al. (2001). Influence of deteriorating ability of emotional comprehension on interpersonal behavior in Alzheimer-yype dementia. *Brain and Cognition, 47,* 423-433. doi: 10.1006/brcg.2001.1318.

Starcevic, V. (2007). Dysphoric about dysphoria: towards a greater conceptual clarity of the term. *Australasian Psychiatry,* 15, 9-12. doi: 10.1080/10398560601083035.

Sunderland, T., Hill, J. L., Lawlor, B. A., & Molchan, S. E. (1988). NIMH Dementia Mood Assessment Scale (DMAS). *Psychopharmacological Bulletin,* 24, 747-753. doi: 10.1017/S1041610297003578.

Vasanthapuram, S. (2011). *Ontology for Psychophysiological Dysregulation of Anger/Aggression.* Available from: http://digitalcommons.unl.edu/computerscidiss/24/.

Visser, P. J., Verhey, F. R., Ponds, R. W., Kester, A., & Jolles, J. (2000). Distinction between preclinical Alzheimer's disease and depression. *Journal of the American Geriatric Society,* 48, 479-484.

Chapter 7: Classification of Behaviors in Dementia/NCDs based on Principles of Compliance and Aggression

Introduction

This chapter focuses on the fourth theoretical construct of behaviors based upon theories of compliance and aggression. Behaviors based in theories of compliance and aggression is seen in an array of mental illnesses varying across the lifespan. The bulk of the understanding of behaviors based in theories of compliance is usually derived from studies in Child and Adolescent developmental psychology. These behaviors, however, are particularly prevalent in adult psychiatry, specifically dementia/NCD and Alzheimer's disease (Benoit et al., 2006). On the other hand, behaviors based in theories of aggression are amongst the most commonly occurring behaviors in patients with dementia/NCD. Aggressive and wandering (agitation) behaviors are the focus of most research and clinical management in dementia/NCD care. Yet there is paucity in the development of new approaches of treatment interventions for these behaviors in patients with dementia/NCD (Benoit et al., 2006).

Behavioral Classification

Two behavioral categories emanating from theories on compliance and aggression, respectively, are:
i.   Oppositional behavior (OB)
ii.   Physically aggressive behaviors (PAB)

Oppositional Behaviors

Items in the oppositional behavior category include:

- Negotiating around care and other needs
- Working against everything the care giver or care provider is attempting with the patient

- Evasive to directions
- Resistive to care, medication or meals or other care directions;
- Barricading and territorialism

Purpose of the Measure

- The purpose of this measure is to make the care giver (CG) or care provider (CP) aware of a bidirectional interaction existing between oneself and the patient.
- Verbal and non-verbal expressions on part of the CG or CP and the patient interact in a dynamic process thereby influencing each other's behaviors.
- CG or CP need to be aware of the impact of their verbal and non-verbal interactions on the existing homeostasis in the patient's environment. Disturbance in homeostasis can occur even when the commands or actions are well intentioned.
- CG or CG needs to be knowledgeable about potential range of non-compliant actions being exhibited by the patient in these circumstances. These actions may range from a patient negotiating to exhibiting passive non-compliance, such as ignoring directions from CG or CP; simple non-compliance, such as a patient hears but refuses to comply without emotional concomitants; to finally showing direct defiance, such as overt refusal with emotional concomitants.
- Each of these individual responses will require a patient centered individualized approach to management.
- Development of care plans which addresses each of the identified level of non-compliance exhibited by the patient. Such an approach will preserve the existing homeostasis in the patient's immediate environment thereby decreasing the probability of emergence of these behaviors.

Specification of the Construct of the Domain

The term "oppositional behaviors" has been used in context of dementia/NCD but has often been categorized with other behaviors such as agitation, psychosis, apathy, and aggression (Ornstein & Gaugler, 2012). An agreed upon specific and concise definition of the construct for oppositional behaviors could not be found in the dementia/NCD literature. Efforts to suggest a definition have been placed forth by Benoit et al. (2006) who describe this behavior as, "refusal by the patient, notably refusal of care, refusal to eat or to cooperate". This definition requires further expansion to explore the depths of the behaviors and thus produce suitable treatment options.

As mentioned in the introduction, there is no agreed upon definition of oppositional behaviors in dementia/NCD literature with the majority currently focusing on child and adolescent psychology. Due to this paucity, review of this construct in child and adolescent developmental psychology was conducted and those principles applied to dementia/NCD care.

Verbal or non-verbal portrayal of "no" in a child's development is seen as an expression of their emerging sense of identity, self-regulation and independence (Greenspan, 1992). Concepts of compliance and non-compliance have been used in context of such interpersonal interactions. These terms have been specifically defined in child developmental psychology. Compliance is defined as, "appropriate following of any instruction to perform a specific response within a reasonable and designate time" (Schoen, 1983). Forehand (1977) proposed the need to separate, "initiation of compliance within a reasonable time after the command is given" and, "completion of the task specified in the command". Forehand and McMahon (1981) defined non-compliance as "refusal to initiate or complete a request made by another person".

There is an interactional process between the person who is giving the command and the person at whom the command is directed. Compliance or non-compliance on part of the person at whom the command is directed is likely to influence the behavior of the person giving the command. Compliance or non-compliance consists of a bidirectional relationship between the two persons thereby forming an interactional unit (Barnett et al., 2012; Kuczynski & Hildebrandt, 1997). This interactional unit forms the conceptual basis to a child's development and sustenance through developmental years.

Kuczynski and Kochanska (1990) have proposed four sub-types of non-compliance, based upon the degree of intellectual functioning and developmental sophistication. The four sub-types include: negotiation, passive non-compliance, simple non-compliance, and direct defiance. In negotiation, the person attempts to modify the nature and conditions of the command (Kuczynski & Kochanska, 1990). Negotiation is seen in persons with higher intellectual functioning and higher levels of developmental sophistication. Negotiation is identified as the most sophisticated strategy in context of interpersonal interactions (Kuczynski & Kochanska, 1990). In passive non-compliance, the person tends not to acknowledge directions given to them (Kuczynski & Kochanska, 1990). In simple non-compliance, the person appears to be acknowledging the commands but refuses to comply and there is no associated hostility or anger (Kuczynski & Kochanska, 1990). Lastly, direct defiance is a variant of non-compliance and is accompanied by hostility and anger (Kuczynski & Kochanska, 1990). Direct defiance is more often observed in persons with lower intellectual functioning.

With increasing cognitive impairment and congruent care needs in persons with dementia/NCD, there is a change in the nature of relationship between the patient and their loved ones. The relationship based in partnership, as is the case in a marriage, starts to change and becomes increasingly dependent in nature. As the degree of dementia/NCD progresses, the dynamic in the relationship becomes increasingly regressive and starts to mirror parent-child relationship. The patient with dementia/NCD is in the child role and the spouse takes on the parental role. In situations with children caring for their parents, there is a reversal in the roles. The patient with dementia/NCD takes on the child like role and the child the parental role.

The bidirectional interactional dynamic proposed by Kuczynski and Hildebrandt (1997) also applies to the relationship between the patient and their partner or patient and their children in its altered format. The patient is in the dependent role and the CG or CP is in the position of giving directions. CG or CP is providing directions and the patient is the one at whom the directions are delivered. This becomes an interactional unit with a bidirectional dynamic. It is the presence of noncompliance in this relationship which forms the basis of oppositional behaviors.

The degree of cognitive impairment the patients exhibits will interact with pre-morbid level of developmental sophistication to give rise to the various sub-types of oppositional behaviors, negotiation, passive non-compliance, simple non-compliance, and direct defiance. In the early stages of cognitive impairment and with a higher level of developmental sophistication, patients will attempt to modify the nature and conditions of the direction. The patient may be seen negotiating around care and other needs. If the patient does not achieve the desired outcome, they may be seen to be working against CG or CP attempts at direction. Passive non-compliance may also be applicable in the early stages of cognitive impairment but with lower levels of developmental sophistication. This will manifest itself as the patient being "evasive to directions".

Simple non-compliance may be applicable in the moderate stages of cognitive impairment and with lower levels of developmental sophistication. This may manifest itself as the patient being "resistive to care, medications or meals or other directions". Direct defiance may be applicable in advanced stages of cognitive impairment and with lower levels of developmental sophistication. Initially, it may present itself as becoming territorial or even barricading oneself in the environment. Continuation of direct defiance to persisting directions can result in Vocal Behaviors (aggressive type) (VB). Further persistence of directions from CG or CP may result in Vocal Behaviors (aggressive type) with associated functional motor activity. Vocal Behaviors (aggressive type) with or without functional motor activity are classified under Emotional Behaviors (Luthra, 2013). On the other hand, continuation of direct defiance to persisting directions may skip the intermediate step of Vocal behaviors (aggressive type) and progress directly to physically aggressive behaviors (PAB). The latter behaviors are classified under *theories on compliance and aggression.* Along this continuum of emergence of behaviors, OB will be the first followed by VB and then finally PAB.

Physically Aggressive Behaviors

Items in the physically aggressive behavior category include:

- Pulling, pushing, grabbing
- Kicking, biting, scratching, punching;
- Spitting, throwing things, breaking objects
- Self-abusive/mutilating behaviors

Purpose of the Measure

- The purpose of this measure is for CG or CP to identify the relationship between the origins of negative emotions, such as anger and discontentment, as a consequence of blockage in goal attainments.

- A perceived discrepancy between the patient and their environment will lead to generation of a need which requires fulfillment. These needs can be physiological, security or belongingness in nature.
- Any perceived impediment by the patient in these needs attainment will result in emergence of negative emotions. As stated earlier and under "emotional behaviors", these responses often tend to be out of proportion in intensity.
- Acts of physical aggression are a sum total of continuation of direct defiance to persistent directions to an out of proportion emotional responses accompanied with functional motor activities. On the other hand, physical aggression can also be the sum total of continuation of direct defiance to persistent direction and perceived impediment to goal attainment of not wanting to change the existing state of homeostasis. CG or CP should make an effort to identify their role or that of the environment to being an impediment to goal attainment for the patient. Behavioral interventions need to be developed around mitigating or eliminating the barriers to goal attainment.

Specification of the Construct of the Category

The definition for "aggression" in relation to dementia/NCD was first defined by Patel and Hope (1992) as, "an overt act, involving the delivery of noxious stimuli to (but not necessarily aimed at) another organism, object or self, which is clearly accidental". Aggressive behaviors have been identified to include physical aggression, aggressive resistance, physical threats, verbal aggression, refusing to speak, destructive behavior, and general irritability (Patel & Hope, 1992). Aggressive behaviors could also be defined to include physical, verbal, or sexual aggression (Patel & Hope, 1992); however, specific types of aggression are not always stipulated within the literature.

Based upon Patel and Hope's (1992) definition, it is not clear if aggressive behavior within dementia/NCD is labeled after the occurrence of one aggressive act or if recurrent acts are required. Cohen-Mansfield's research on agitation in dementia/NCD patients defines aggression as a component of agitation (Buhr & White, 2006). Evidence has been presented regarding perception of care providers as to which behaviors are considered to be aggressive, is a subjective and not always reliable statement (Pulsford & Duxbury, 2006). Physical aggressive behaviors (PAB) are one of the most frequently occurring behaviors in patients with dementia/NCDs (Dennehy et al., 2013). It is also the most frequently documented behaviors associated with high risks. In fact it is so much so that PAB form the basis for all involuntary admissions to acute mental health facilities.

A review of psychology literature provides a rather heterogeneous conceptual approach to understanding the construct of aggression. These different angles used to define the construct of aggression are as follows:

- The biological perspective of aggression focuses on the genetic predisposition and changes in physiological functioning as the basis to generation of aggression. Various disease states may cause a change in brain function by producing changes in neurotransmitter functioning as the basis for aggression

- The behavioral perspective of aggression focuses on the principles of Classical and Operant conditioning as the basis for aggression. The behavior of aggression is viewed as a learned behavior and there are variables in the milieu which either reinforce them or attenuate them
- The cognitive perspective of aggression focuses on the mechanics of mental processing of information (information processing module; IPM) for the basis of aggression. Impairment in cognitive functions of memory, thinking, language, problem-solving and decision making form the basis of emergence of aggression
- The evolutionary perspective of aggression focuses on the role of aggression in evolution of homo sapiens to their present day status. Buss and Shackelford (1997) viewed aggression as a solution to a particular adaptive problem and one example of such an adaptive problem is "defense against attack". According to the evolutionary view, the primary role of aggression is to aid in survival and reproduction
- The cross-cultural perspective focuses on how different cultures influence our perspective regarding aggressive behaviors. It also helps understand cultural difference in frequency of such behaviors as well

It is important to note that all above perspectives are not mutually exclusive of each other but rather co-exist in a complementary manner. All of these perspectives need to be applied to any given patient exhibiting aggressive behaviors to fully elucidate an understanding of the patient specific response and appropriate management thereof.

Aggression is further classified into two distinct categories: instrumental and hostile aggression (Siegel & Victoroff, 2009). Instrumental aggression is based in a reward-consequence paradigm. It proposes there is a process of systematic thinking involved in evaluating the benefits or rewards of aggression, referred to as "aggression pays". Likewise, as the benefits or rewards are withdrawn, the aggression will subside.

Hostile aggression is based in emotional responses to provocation or negative feelings. Dollard et al.(1939) put forth the "frustration-aggression theory" as the way to explain the aggression based in "provocation". According to Dollard et al. (1939), an individual perceiving any kind of a block towards accomplishing their goal will become provoked and subsequently frustrated. This will lead to an act of aggression. Hence, it is an external interference to accomplishing of goals which leads to frustration and ultimately aggression. (Berkowitz, 1989) put forth a much broader model to explain aggression based in negative feelings. According to (Berkowitz, 1989) any/all underlying causes of negative feelings can lead to aggression. The underlying causes can have their basis in biological, psychological or social perturbations (Dettmore, Kolanowski & Boustani, 2009).

Hence, when evaluating aggression in patients with dementia/NCD the following approach should be taken:

- Assess the aggressive act from various perspectives (biological, behavioral, cognitive, evolutionary and cross-cultural) to understand the occurrence in that moment in time and in that particular context

- Assess if the act falls under the instrumental or hostile category. One would hope that almost all acts of aggression in patients with dementia/NCDs fall under the hostile category
- If the act of aggression falls under the instrumental category, a careful assessment of the patient's ability to understand and appreciate the foreseeable consequences of their act needs to be conducted immediately. Depending upon the outcome of this assessment, appropriate treatment and safety interventions need to be put in place and in accordance with the local legal jurisdictions
- If the act of aggression falls under the "hostile" category, an attempt should be made to identify which specific goal attainment was blocked or the basis of these underlying negative feeling

Conclusions

The nature of relationship between patients with progressive cognitive impairment and CGs changes over the duration of the decline. This presents as a role reversal, as is the case between children and their parents with dementia/NCD, or regression to parent-child (as is the case between partners) in the nature of relationships. This bidirectional interactional unit develops a level of homeostasis for its sustenance. Variables, which either destabilize this homeostasis or impede in goal attainment will give rise to behaviors in this category. For both oppositional and aggressive behaviors, focus should be placed on identification of these variables and care plans developed and utilized to mitigate the effect of these variables as a way to managing behaviors.

References

Barnett, M.A., Gustafsson, H., Deng, M., Mills-Koonce, W.R., & Cox, M. (2012). Bidirectional associations among sensitive parenting, language development, and social competence. *Infant and Child Development*, 21, 374-393. doi: 10.1002/icd.1750.

Benoit, M. et al. (2006). Professional consensus on the treatment of agitation, aggressive behaviour, oppositional behaviour and psychotic disturbances in dementia. *The journal of nutrition, health & aging*, 10, 410-415.

Berkowitz, L. (1989). Frustration-aggression hypothesis: Examination and reformulation. *Psychological Bulletin*, 106, 59-73. doi: 10.1037/0033-2909.106.1.59.

Buhr, G. T., & White, H. K. (2006). Difficult behaviors in long-term care patients with dementia. *Journal of the American Medical Directors Association*, 7, 180-192. doi: 10.1016/j.jamda.2006.12.012.

Buss, D. M., & Shackelford, T. K. (1997). Human aggression in evolutionary psychological perspective. *Clinical Psychology Review*, 17, 605-619. doi: 10.1016/S0272-7358(97)00037-8.

Davis, L. L., Buckwalter, K., & Burgio, L. D. (1997). Measuring problem behaviors in dementia: developing a methodological agenda. *Advances in Nursing Science*, 20, 40-55.

Dennehy, E. B., Kahle-Wrobleski, K., Sarsour, K., & Milton, D. R. (2013). Derivation of a brief measure of agitation and aggression in Alzheimer's disease. *International Journal of Geriatric Psychiatry*, 28, 182–189. doi: 10.1002/gps.3807.

Dettmore, D., Kolanowski, A., & Boustani, M. (2009). Aggression in persons with dementia: use of nursing theory to guide clinical practice. *Geriatric Nursing*, 30, 8-17. doi: 10.1016/j.gerinurse.2008.03.001.

Dollard, J., Doob, L. W., Miller, N. E., Mowrer, O. H., & Sears, R. R. (1939). *Frustration and aggression.* New Haven: Yale University Press.

Forehand, R. (1977). Child noncompliance to prenatal requests: Behavioral analysis and treatment. In M. Hersen, M. Eisler, & P. M. Miller (Eds.), *Progress in behavior modification* (pp. 111-148). Sand Diego: Academic Press.

Forehand, R. L., & McMahon, R. J. (1981). *Helping the noncompliant child: A clinician's guide to parent training.* New York: Guilford Press.

Greenspan, S.I. (1992). *Infancy and Early Childhood: The Practice of Clinical Assessment and Intervention with Emotional and Developmental Challenges.* Madison: International Universities Press.

Kuczynski, L., & Hildebrandt, N. (1997). Models of conformity and resistance in socialization theory. In J. E. Grusec, & L. Kuczynski (Eds.), *Parenting and children's internalization of values: A handbook of contemporary theory.* (pp. 227-256). Hoboken: Johen Wiley & Sons.

Kuczynski, L., & Kochanska, G. (1990). Development of children's noncompliance strategies from toddlerhood to age 5. *Developmental Psychology*, 26, 398-408.

Luthra, A.S. (2013). *New Terminology to Label Behaviors in Dementias: Stage Congruent Responsive Behaviors (SCRB).* Manuscript submitted for publication.

Luthra, A.S. (2013). *Classification of behaviors in dementiabased in impairment in theories based upon information processing pathways.* Manuscript submitted for publication.

Luthra, A.S. (2013). *Classification of Behaviors in Dementia based in "motivational" and "needs based" theories.* Manuscript submitted for publication.

Luthra, A.S. (2013). *Classification of behaviors in Dementias based upon theories of regulation of emotions.* Manuscript submitted for publication.

Ornstein, K., & Gaugler, J. E. (2012). The problem with "problem behaviors": a systematic review of the association between individual patient behavioral and psychological symptoms and caregiver depression and burden within the dementia patient–caregiver dyad. *International Psychogeriatrics*, 24, 1536-1552. doi: 10.1017/S1041610212000737.

Patel, V. & Hope, R.A. (1992) A rating scale for aggressive behaviour in the elderly - the RAGE. *Psychological medicine*, 22, 211-221.

Siegel, A., & Victoroff, J. (2009). Understanding human aggression: new insights from neuroscience. *International journal of law and psychiatry*, 32, 209-215. doi: 10.1016/j.ijlp.2009.06.001.

Schoen, S. F. (1983). The status of compliance technology: Implications for programming. *The Journal of Special Education*, 17, 483-496. doi: 10.1177/002246698301700410.

World Health Organization. (2012). *World Alzheimer Report 2012, A public health priority.* Available from: http://whqlibdoc.who.int/publications/2012/9789241564458_eng.pdf

Chapter 8: Classification of Behaviors in the Heterogeneous Group: Vocal and Sexual Behaviors in Patients with Dementia/NCD

Introduction

This chapter focuses on the final group of behavioral categories which require a combination of theoretical constructs to justify their occurrence. The two behavioral categories emanating in this group are:

1. Vocal Behaviors
2. Sexual Behaviors

It becomes rather apparent from review of the literature there is vast heterogeneity in the clinical presentation of these behavioral symptoms in patterns with advanced dementia. Multiple proposed classification systems on VB and SB have been put forth in the literature; as will become evident in the following paragraphs. No single "specification of the construct" identified in this book could explain for the occurrence of these heterogeneous behaviors. Hence, there was a need to utilize all the identified "specification of the constructs" to explain for the presence of these behavioral categories.

Vocal Behaviors

Vocal behaviors (VB) present as one of the most challenging in patients with dementia/NCD (Von Gunten et al., 2008). Management of VB in clinical practice is extremely frustrating and are amongst the most likely of the behaviors responsible caregiver (CG) or care provider (CP) distress (Teresi et al., 1997).

Various efforts have to date made attempts to classify and understand VB. For example, Ryan et al (1988), Cohen-Mansfield and Werner (1997), Magri et al (2007) have attempted to present a classification of VB and the following is a brief review of highlights from their findings.

Ryan et al. (1988) have proposed six subtypes of VB:

1. Noise making which appears purposeless and repetitive
2. Noise making in response to the environment
3. Noise making which elicits a response from the environment
4. "Chatterbox" noise making
5. Noise making due to deafness
6. Other noise making.

Cohen-Mansfield and Werner (1997) put forth an alternative way of classifying VB referred to as *typology of vocalizations* (TOV). This classification was designed to assist in better understanding of the meaning of VB. Four dimensions on which these behaviors were classified were:

1. Type of sound
2. Purpose of sound including response to the environment
3. Timing, including frequency and pattern of occurrence
4. Level of disruptiveness (Cohen-Mansfield & Werner, 1997)

Magri, Ferry & Abela (2007) summarized all the above variables into four sub-headings to include:

i.   VB due to physical illness (unmet physiological needs)
ii. VB due to underlying psychiatric illness (depression, anxiety, psychosis, impulse dyscontrol,
iii. VB due to underlying personality
iv. VB due to environment (under or over stimulation and caregiver behaviors)

Attempts to better understand VB have also been pursued by associating the behaviors with different parts of the brain; mostly frontal lobe or interruption of fronto-subcortical circuits (Nagaratnam, Patel & Whelan, 2003) and abnormalities in neuron-chemical substrates such as serotonergic dysfunction (Greenwald, Marin & Silverman, 1986; Dwyer & Byrne 2000). Attempts have been made to link VB with underlying psychiatric illnesses such as depression; psychosis; underlying personality; disruption of impulse control; unmet physiological needs or linking them to environmental factors such as "over-stimulation", "under-stimulation", and caregiver behaviors. (Cohen-Mansfield, Werner & Marx, 1990; Dwyer & Byrne 2000 and Margi, Ferry & Abela, 2007).

Yet another variable influencing VB is impairment in language functions. Matteau et al. (2003) reported an increased prevalence of VB in patients with altered language functions in comparison to those with preserved language abilities. Additionally, clinical anecdotal experience seems to point to an increased prevalence of VB in patients with impaired mobility. Unfortunately, there is paucity of published literature to either support or discount this clinical observation.

All of the existing classifications of VB fail to assist health care professional and family members, alike, in understanding the "meaning" or the "purpose" of VB from the patient's point of view. The proposed new classification makes an attempt to accomplish this desired goal.

New Proposed Classification of VB

In an effort to classify VB, it soon became apparent there was no single "specification of the construct" which could assist in understanding the basis or meaning for the occurrence of these behaviors. Classifications of VB based in various "Specification of the Construct" are as follows:

I.   VB based in theories of regulation of emotions
II.   VB based in theories of motivation and needs based
        a.   VB based in Goal-Directed Cognitions (GDC)
        b.   VB based in Importuning Behaviors (IB)
III. VB based in theories of self-stimulation

Hence, the final classification of VB includes five (5) subtypes:

I.   VB Aggressive type
II.   VB Effusive type
III. VB Based in Goal Directed Cognitions (GDC)
IV.   VB based in Importuning and/or Fretfulness
V.   VB based in Self Stimulation

Items in the Vocal Behavior Category Include:

- Explosive, Argumentative and Quarrelsome
- Talking loud and fast, acting "manic-like"
- Yelling and screaming to get things done
- Rattling bed rails/table tops, persistent calling out for staff, family or "parents"
- Making any kind of strange noises or repetitious sounds

Purpose of the Measure or Meaning of the Behaviors

Recognition of behaviors in this category is to make the care givers and providers aware of a complex, multifaceted, basis of their occurrence in patients with dementia/NCD. It could represent any one of the following:

Explosiveness, Argumentative, and Quarrelsome

These behavioral symptoms represent the expression of the primary emotions of irritability and discontentment. These symptoms are included under the category of VB aggressive type. Recognition of behaviors in this category is to make CG and CP aware of the defensive and attack nature of interactions by the patients in their immediate environment. The purpose of the "defensive" mode, for the patient, is to prevent further exposure to a perceived noxious stimulus in their immediate environment. These behaviors take the form of explosiveness. These behaviors are to be viewed by CG or CP as a "shot across the bow'" by the patient. CG or CP should heed to this warning signal and attempt to identify possible triggers in the immediate milieu as being contributory. These triggers will need to be extinguished to prevent further escalation in behaviors. Continued presence of these perceived noxious stimuli runs the risk of pushing the behavior into an "attack" mode. These behaviors may take the form of becoming argumentativeness and quarrelsome. Continued escalation of these behaviors may result in physical aggression directed towards the noxious stimuli. These behaviors should also alert the CG or CP to the "out of proportion'" responses of dementia/NCD patients to various perceived noxious stimuli. When attempting to interact with dementia/NCD patients under these circumstances, CG or CP should make an effort to calibrate their own emotional responses such that patient's behaviors do not get pushed from a "defensive" to an "attack" mode.

Talking Fast and Loud, Acting Manic-like

These behavioral symptoms represent the expression of the primary emotion of happiness. These symptoms are included under the category of VB effusive type. Recognition of symptoms in this category is to make CG or CP aware of the excitable and "out of proportion" responses of dementia/NCD patients to pleasant stimuli in their environment. CG and CP should make an effort to create a low stimulation environment to diminish the "out of proportion" responses in such circumstances. When attempting to interact with dementia/NCD patients under these circumstances, CG or CP should make an effort to calibrate their own emotional responses such that patient's behaviors do not escalate any further. This is because CG or CP need to remain cognizant of the risks associated with these 'out of proportion" responses to pleasurable stimuli in the environment. Amongst the risk identified is the emergence of sexual behaviors or emotional instability leading to verbal and/or physical aggression.

Yelling and Screaming To Get Things Done (In Their Environment)

These behavioral symptoms are under the category of VB based in GDC. Recognition of behaviors in this category is to ensure care givers (CG) or care providers (CP) are aware of the "busy beaver" like states in patients with dementia/NCD. These symptoms are reflective of the "busy" state of the patients mind. These patients tend to be very persistent with their demands and actions thereby creating a very high energy environment.

When a patient perceives a discrepancy between their internal state and a stimulus in their milieu, it forms the basis of triggering a "need" which requires fulfilment. Motivational forces propel the patient to satiate these "needs". The degree of activation of motivational forces generated will determine whether the needs are expressed as "thoughts" or "action". The majority of patients exhibiting VB (GDC), though not everyone, tend to be demented with concurrent immobility. Their immobility makes it difficult to satiate identified needs through actions. Hence, they seem to be directing care givers and care providers to satiate needs on their behalf. Behaviors in this category are the result of heightened motivational drives due to the disease state of dementia/NCD.

The specific need requiring fulfilment by these behaviors is that of "belongingness". The "belongingness" need encompasses being affiliated or accepted by ones milieu or environment, working towards and meeting one's obligations and responsibilities in order to be a part of larger society or milieu.

Hence, the locus of control for these needs underlying the genesis of GDC or GDA tends to be external to the patient and the triggers are present in their immediate external environment.

If the "busy" states involve thinking and as is the case in these set of behaviors, patients are repeatedly coming up with directives or requesting specific things they require done in their environment. GDC are activation of specific mental schemas in the brain from triggers in the external environment. As long as those triggers remain constant in the milieu, GDC persist. (Refer to article on "behaviors based in theories of information processing" for detailed information on this construct).

Rattling Bed Rails/Table Tops, Persistent Calling Out for Staff, Family or "Parents"

These behavioral symptoms can either represent fulfilment of "physiological" or "security" needs. Please refer to chapter 4 (Behavioral classification based on motivational and needs-based theories) under the Importuning category for understanding of meaning of behaviors fulfilling "physiological" needs. Please refer to chapter 5 (Behavioral classification based on theories of regulation of emotions) under the Fretful/Trepidated category for understanding of behaviors fulfilling "security" needs.

Making Strange Noises and Making Repetitive Sounds

These behavioral symptoms represent a feeling of being "detached" or "disconnected" from their immediate environment. This is particularly valid in dementia/NCD patients who tend to be immobile or less mobile and suffer further sensory deprivation such as visual or hearing impairment. All the approach needs to be directed towards "connecting" these patients to their environment. Hence, multi-sensory stimulation techniques, through the use of Snoozelin Room and Montessori methods, can be very helpful in achieving that "connectedness" for the patient.

Specification of the Construct of the Category

VB based in Aggressiveness and/or Effusiveness

Please refer to Chapter 5 *Classification of Behaviors based upon Theories of Emotional Regulation* for details on the "Specification of the Construct" for "aggressiveness" or "effusiveness".

VB based in Goal-Directed Cognitions

Please refer to chapter 4 titled *Classification of Behaviors based in Motivation and Needs-Based Theories* for details on the Specification of the Construct" for "goal-directed cognitions.

VB Based in Importuning and/or Fretfulness

Please refer to chapter 4 titled Classification of Behaviors based in Motivation and Needs-Based Theories and chapter 5 titled Classification of Behaviors based upon Theories of Emotional Regulation for details on "Specification of Constructs" for "Importuning" and "fretfulness", respectively.

VB Based in Theories on Self-stimulatory (SS)

The majority of the understanding on SS behaviors comes from literature on Autism. In dementia/NCD literature, the term SS behaviors have been used in context of wandering (Lai & Arthur, 2002), noise making (Lai, 1999) and sexual behaviors (Connor, Burgio & Butler, 1987). Wandering behaviors are those most referenced in association with SS behaviors (Lai & Arthur, 2002).

Several authors (Baumiester & Forehand, 1973; Green 1967; Green, 1968; Cleland & Clark, 1966) have hypothesised that a certain level of stimulation in tactile, vestibular and kinaesthetic modalities is necessary for the organism, in a given environment, to stay connected with the environment. "Sense" is any faculty by which stimuli from outside or inside the body are received and felt. Such faculties include hearing, sight, smell, touch, taste and equilibrium. "Perception" is the feeling produced by the stimulus. Vestibular apparatus is situated in the inner ear and is responsible for detecting changes in speed and direction of head movements. Vestibular system operates in conjunction with visual and proprioceptive systems to maintain a state of equilibrium in an individual. Proprioception refers to "perception of one's own self" as opposed to kinaesthetic which refers to "sense of body's motion or movement". Kinaesthetic modality is that sense which detects the bodily position, weight or movements of the muscles, joints and tendons. Kinaesthetic sense is differentiated from proprioceptive sense by excluding the sense of equilibrium or balance. In addition to maintaining equilibrium, vestibular system also serves the purpose of directing the gaze of eyes and a line of vision (eyes are connected to the ears).

If the level of stimulation in any of the above modalities is insufficient, the organism may engage in activities or behaviors to compensate for that deficiency and as a means of providing itself with that added level of sensory stimulation. In a given environment, a patient with cognitive impairment will develop a state of homeostasis in its level of stimulation in the three modalities (tactile, vestibular and kinaesthetic), between itself and the environment. Added sensory impairment in any of the perceptions and inclusive of auditory, visual, olfactory, gustatory or tactile will further add to the imbalance in the state of homeostasis in those three modalities (tactile, vestibular and kinaesthetic). Any further changes in the environment (milieu structure or interpersonal interactions) or the patient's internal factors (innate physiological needs and Circadian Rhythms) which result in the level of stimulation to drop below a certain "threshold" can theoretically generate behaviors to compensate for that loss (Luthra, 2013). VB would be one such manifestation of SS behaviors. Otherwise, VB based in SS is a diagnosis of exclusion. In any patient presenting with VB, all other subtype of VB have to be ruled out first before the VB can be labelled as based in SS.

If the VB are identified to be based in any of the other subtypes, aforementioned non-pharmacological approaches need to be implemented in these patients with a view to mitigating associate risks. If all such interventions fail, an attempt needs to be made to do a detailed search of variables which may be contributory to changes in level of stimulation in tactile, vestibular or kinaesthetic modalities of the patient. Once identified, medical and non-medical interventions need to be put in place to compensate for diminished level of stimulation in that particular modality to re-establish a state of homeostasis. According to Magri, Ferry and Abela (2007), any of the following interventions, either singularly or in combination, may be used to re-established the homeostasis amongst the modalities; use a calm, unhurried approach; use a warm reassuring voice; emphasize non-verbal communications and eye contact; explain procedures/happenings; implement void expression of judgemental thoughts and feelings; reduce meaningless excessive stimuli e.g. noise, TV, high traffic areas; relieve immediate discomforts; provide orientation cues; and provide meaningful activity.

Sexual Behaviors (SB)

The expression of sexual behavior by persons with dementia/NCD poses a unique spectrum of challenges for care providers (Mahieu & Gastmans, 2012). On one end of the spectrum lays the normal and healthy progression of human sexuality that grows well into late adulthood, while on the other end lays the challenge of the impact of dementia/NCD on this otherwise normal process. Whereas, the overt set of sexual behaviors poses a greater challenge during direct patient care, the near-normal expression of sexuality presents the truly probing question of when to label them as pathological (Mahieu & Gastmans, 2012). This clinical situation is further complicated by stigmatization and a biased understanding of what indeed constitutes a normal expression of sexuality in dementia/NCD population (Mahieu & Gastmas, 2012). Amongst other questions to be pondered are; whether a particular act is appropriate or inappropriate and how does one define appropriateness?, whether the behavior arises from malicious intent or as a result of the illness?, and finally, if an act of sexual behavior occurs, was it even a sexual act in the first place, or was it just perceived as such by care providers?

Whereas, the last two decades have witnessed an explosion of literature on this topic, there is paucity of articles which can find a common ground in the understanding of the use of terminology, definitions, classification and diagnostic criteria of sexual behaviors in patients with dementia/NCD (Mahieu & Gastmans, 2012). Varying ideas also exist with regards to the mechanisms which underlay the occurrence of these behaviors and inclusive of biological, psychosocial, and environmental mechanisms. Further, researchers and care providers acknowledge the need for further research in this domain (Mahieu & Gastmans, 2012).

Various terms used to describe such behaviors in patients with dementia/NCD include Inappropriate Sexual Behavior (ISB), Hypersexuality, Sexual Disinhibition, Inappropriate Sexual Expression, Aberrant Sexual Behavior (Kuhn, Grenier & Arseneau, 1998; Johnson, Knight, & Alderman, 2006). In this paper, we will use the term "sexual behaviors" (SB) so as not to engage in the discussions over "appropriateness or inappropriateness" which is often fraught with elements of judgment and biases. The term SB does not imply that other terms are unsuitable for use in clinical practice.

Definitions of these terms are also as varied as the terminologies. "Inappropriate sexual behavior is a problem behavior symptomatic of dementia/NCD. Hypersexuality is not deliberate behavior... Hypersexuality is not a form of sexual intimacy that may be retained in AD. The nurse must assess this behavior as either retained sexual intimacy or as problem behavior. Retained sexual intimacy is appropriate sexual behaviors that occur in the wrong place" Robinson (2003). Hypersexuality was outlined by Kuhn, Grenier & Arseneau (1998) as the following: "Hypersexuality is not to be confused with responsible forms of sexual intimacy that may be diminished, retained, or renewed in the course of AD." Alagiakrishnan et al. (2005) defines abnormal sexual behavior as, "unwanted sexual advances such as climbing into bed with other residents in a nursing home or actual attempts of intercourse and aberrant sexual behavior such as sexual aggression." Likewise, classification of SB is also rather varied as well. According to Szasz (1983) and Tucker (2010), inappropriate sexual behaviors have been divided into three types:

i.   Sex talk: using foul language that is not in keeping with a patient's premorbid personality

ii.   Sexual acts: touching, grabbing, exposing or masturbating in public or private places

iii.   Implied sexual acts: openly reading pornographic material or requesting unnecessary genital care

An alternative way to classify SB was placed forth by de Medeiros et al. (2008); this way of classifying divided improper sexual behaviors into two types:

i.   Intimacy seeking, referring to normal behaviors that are misplaced in social context (kissing, hugging)

ii.   Disinhibited, referring to rude and intrusive behaviors that would be considered inappropriate in most contexts (lewdness, fondling, and exhibitionism)

The only validated scale for classifying and measuring severity of ISB is St Andrews Sexual Behavior Assessment (SASBA) (Stubbs, 2011). SASBA was developed at St Andrews Health-care in the United Kingdom by Knight et al. (2008).

There are several issues arising from review of the literature which need stating and require further discussion.

What Defines "Inappropriateness"?

Literature has extensively grappled with this issue and no consensus has been achieved. As an example; literature considers "excessive hugging and kissing" as ISB (Alkhalil et al., 2004) while others have labeled "urination or defecation in public" as ISB (Howell & Watts, 1990). The list of symptoms labeled as ISB is rather exhaustive. Based upon the research conducted by Howell and Watts (1990), Kuhn, Grenier and Arseneau (1998), Robinson (2003), Hajjard and Kamel (2004), Tucker (2010), and Alkhalil et al. (2004), list of behaviors labeled as ISB are as follows:

i.   Disrobing in Public

ii.   Masturbating in Public

iii.   Increase or Decrease in Libido
iv.   Inappropriate Sexual Advances
v.   Sexually Demanding/Aggressiveness
vi.   Lewd/Suggestive/Foul Language
vii.   Fondling Self/Another
viii.   Flirtatious Behavior
ix.   Viewing Pornography
x.   Sexual Preoccupation
xi.   Delusions of Spouse's Infidelity

As stated earlier, there is ambiguity in the use of these terms and where do clinicians draw a line on the threshold between acts of normal sexual growth and expression and dementia/NCD-related sexual behavior? This issue has been repeatedly debated in the literature (Johnson, Knight, & Alderman, 2006; Rheaume & Mitty, 2008; Wallace & Safer, 2009; Elias & Ryan, 2010; Stubbs, 2011). It is imperative for the CG and CP to have sufficient knowledge about the patient's sexuality prior to developing dementia/NCD in order to fully appreciate the impact of labeling behaviors as ISB (Tucker, 2010).

Role of Environment in Labeling of SB

The environment plays a substantial role in complicating the definitions around ISB. Several authors (Rheaume & Mitty, 2008; Wallace & Safer, 2009; Elias & Ryan, 2011) have stated that an expression of human sexuality may be perfectly normal in the privacy of one's bedroom and the labeling of "abnormality" is rather the phenomenon of setting in which the behavior is occurring. As an example, the act of masturbation in privacy of a room would be labeled as a normal expression of sexuality but when done anywhere outside that privacy gets labeled "abnormal". Therefore, is it really a problem of expression of patient's sexuality or a problem of being unaware of their environment and loss of self-monitoring? (Benbow & Beeston, 2012). The same argument can be extended to a patient who misidentifies another patient or staff member as their spouse and makes sexual advances. In this situation, an otherwise normal expression of sexuality may get labeled as ISB (Benbow & Beeston, 2012).

The second environmental factor to be considered is that of differing social, moral and religious values amongst various care providers in the institution or in the society-at-large. A simple example of this would be that of a married couple showing affection in public, where one of the spouses has dementia/NCD, labeled as ISB by staff who witnesses the act? It may be reasonable to extrapolate from this example that many reported "incidents" of ISB are indeed the result of labeling of behaviors by staff when applying their own value systems to the situation and not evaluating the situation objectively (Benbow & Beeston, 2012). A similar argument could be applied to dementia/NCD patients who are primarily seeking a connection with another human being or some form of sensory stimulation as ISB when it had no bearing on that patient's expression of their sexuality, whatsoever (Kuhn, Greiner & Arseneau, 1998). These behaviors represent the primary human need for "intimacy" and to paraphrase Kuhn, Greiner & Arseneau (1998) "Behavior of people with dementia/NCD may be misconstrued as sexual in nature when, in fact, it may have an entirely different purpose or meaning… The person with AD may not be thinking "sex" at all as much as expressing a desire to feel connected to another person, albeit in a personal and physical way. Whether a hand, shoulder, or breast is being touched may be irrelevant to the person with dementia/NCD. However, this behavior may be interpreted as sexually explicit and inappropriate by others".

New Proposed Classification of SB

In an effort to classify SB, it soon became apparent there was no single "specification of the construct" could assist us in understanding the heterogeneous basis of these behaviors. In order to accommodate such heterogeneity, "Specification of the Construct' based in theories of *information processing, motivation and needs-based* and on *regulation of emotions* have been all been used to classify SB and as follows:

I.   SB based in theories of information processing
     a.   SB based in over-identification of visual facial stimuli. This will result in Misplace Intimacy (MI).
     b.   SB based in Attribution Error (mislabelling patient's actions) (AE)
II.   SB based in theories on motivation and needs-based
     a.   SB based in Stimulus Bound Behaviors (SBB)
     b.   SB based in Importuning Behaviors (IB)
III.   SB based in theories on regulation of emotions
     a.   SB based innate need for intimacy (INI) or a "secure base"

Hence, the final classification of SB includes:

I.   SB based in MI
II.   SB based in AE
III.   SB based in SBB
IV.   SB based in IB
V.   SB based in INI

Items in the sexual behavior category include:

- Verbally Sexual (Comments, Gestures, Innuendos)
- Physically Sexual (Grabbing breasts, buttocks, crotch)
- Self-Stimulation (masturbating)

Purpose of the Measure or Meaning of the Behaviors

Recognition of behaviors in this category is to make the care givers and providers aware of a complex, multifaceted, basis of their occurrence in patients with dementia/NCD. It could represent any one of the following:

- SB based in MI and AE. This category of behaviors is to make care giver (CG) and care providers (CP) aware of the potential of mislabelling of behaviors. In the case of MI, the patient is over identifying another patient as their spouse and expressing appropriate affection. This SB is based in over-identification of visual facial stimuli. In the case of SB based in AE, it can be reported by another co-patient or observed by the staff. If reported by another co-patient, it is to make CG and CP cognizant of the role of one's own moral and religious values in labelling of behaviors. The fundamental attribution error refers to the systematic bias that individuals draw inferences or conclusions from previous knowledge (Tetlock, 1985).
- SB based in SBB and IB. This category of behaviors is to make CG and CP aware of:

    i.   Impairment of self-awareness and monitoring
    ii.   Need to fulfil basic "physiological needs"

SB based in SBB is to make CG and CP aware of the loss a patient's ability to be aware of the social inappropriateness of their actions in the immediate social context. SB based in IB is to make CG and CP aware of the preservation of innate physiological needs well into the very late stages of dementia/NCD.

- SB based in INI. This category of behaviors is to make CG and CP aware of the need of the patient to feel secure in their environment through connection with other human beings.
- Behavioral care planning needs to be specific to each of the above set of circumstances.

Specification of the Construct of the Category

SB based in MI and A

Please refer to the original article titled "Classification of behaviors in dementia/NCD based in impairment in theories based upon information processing pathways" for details on this "Specification of Constructs" (Luthra, 2013).

VB based in SBB and IB

By definition, these behaviors are specifically tied to an overt or an obvious stimulus and persist as long as the stimulus persists. Once the stimulus is removed, the behavior ceases to exist (Luthra, 2013). Physiological or psychological deficiencies may be trigged by external or internal stimuli, generating a need that requires fulfillment (Luthra, 2013). These needs tend be physiological, security, or belongingness in nature in patients with even advanced stages of dementia/NCD. If the stimulus is not removed, the patient will attempt to fulfill the need by engaging in sexually inappropriate behavior (Luthra, 2013). However, once or if the stimulus is removed, the inappropriate sexual behavior ceases to exist (Luthra, 2013). Please refer to the original article titled *Classification of Behaviors based in Motivation and Needs-Based Theories* for additional details on this "Specification of Constructs" (Luthra, 2013).

VB based in INI

Please refer to the original article titled Classification of Behaviors based in Motivation and Needs-Based Theories and Classification of Behaviors based upon Theories of Emotional Regulation for details on this "Specification of Constructs" (Luthra, 2013; Luthra, 2013).

Conclusions

VB and SB are amongst the most complex behaviors in patients with dementia/NCD. There is no singular way of understanding the occurrence of these behaviors. Several of the "Specification of the Construct" has been utilized to classify VB and SB. Subtypes of VB include aggressive type, effusive type, those based in goal-directed cognitions, fretful and/or importuning and self-stimulatory type. Subtypes of SB include those based in misplaced intimacy, attribution error, stimulus bound, importuning and innate need for intimacy. An approach to evaluating VB and SB with conscious recognition of such a heterogeneity of causes for their presence should lead to more comprehensive understanding. This, in turn, should lead to more innovative non-pharmacological interventions and judicious use of pharmacology.

References

Alagiakrishnan, K., et al. (2005). Sexually inappropriate behaviour in demented elderly people. *Postgraduate medical journal, 81*(957), 463-466.

Alkhalil, C., Tanvir, F., Alkhalil, B., & Lowenthal, D. T. (2004). Treatment of sexual disinhibition in dementia: case reports and review of the literature. *American Journal of Therapetuics,* 11, 231-235.

Benbow, S. M., & Beeston, D. (2012). Sexuality, aging, and dementia. *International Psychogeriatrics*, 24, 1-8. doi: 10.1017/S1041610212000257.

Baumiester, AA. & Forehand, R. (1973) Stereotyped acts in N.R. Ellis (Ed). International review of research in mental retardation. (Vol 6). *New York Academic Press.*

Cleland, CC. & Clark, CM. (1966) Sensory deprivation and aberrant behavior among idiots. *American Journal of mental deficiency*, 71, 213-225. Cohen-Mansfield & Werner, P. (1997) Topoly of disruptive vocalization in older persons suffering from dementia. *International Journal of Geriatric Psychiatry*, 12, 1079-1091. doi: 10.1002/(SICI)1099-1166(199711)12;11<1079::AID-GPS689>3.0.CO;2-P.

Conn, D., & Thorpe, L. (2007). Assessment of behavioural and psychological symptoms associated with dementia. *The Canadian Journal of Neurological Sciences, 34*, S67-S71.

Connor, A.B., Burgio, LD., Butler, F. (1987) An observational analysis of self-stimulatory behaviors of older adults in a nursing home: Behavioural interventions, 2, 189-197. doi: 10.1002/bin.2360020402.

Davis, L.L., Buckwalter, K. & Burgio, L.D. (1997). Measuring problem behaviors in dementia: Developing a methodological agenda. *Advances in Nursing Science*, 20, 40-55.

Davis, T. R., & Luthans, F. (1980). A social learning approach to organizational behavior. *Academy of Management Review*, *5*(2), 281-290.

de Medeiros, K., Rosenberg, P. B., Baker, A. S., & Onyike, C. U. (2008). Improper sexual behaviors in elders with dementia living in residential care. *Dementia and Geriatric Cognitive Disorders*, 26, 370-377. doi: 10.1159/000163219.

Dwyer, M., & Byrne, G. J. (2000). Disruptive vocalization and depression in older nursing home residents. *International Psychogeriatrics*, 12, 463-471. doi: 10.1017/S104161020000658X.

Elias, J., & Ryan, A. (2010). A review and commentary on the factors that influence expressions of sexuality by older people in care homes. *Journal of Clinical Nursing*, 20, 1668-1676. doi: 10.1111/j.1365-2702.2010.03409.x.

Finkel, S. I., Costa e Silva, J., Cohen, G., Miller, S., & Sartorius, N. (1997). Behavioral and psychological signs and symptoms of dementia: a consensus statement on current knowledge and implications for research and treatment.*International Psychogeriatrics*, *8*(S3), 497-500.

Forehand, R. (1977). Child noncompliance to prenatal requests: Behavioral analysis and treatment. In M. Hersen, M. Eisler, & P. M. Miller (Eds.), *Progress in behavior modification* (Vol. 5, pp. 111-148). Sand Diego: Academic Press.

Forehand, R. L., & McMahon, R. J. (1981). *Helping the noncompliant child: A clinician's guide to parent training.* New York: Guilford Press.

Green, A.H. (1967) Self-mutilation in Schizophrenic children. *Archives of General Psychiatry*, 17, 234-244. doi: 10.1001/archpsyc.1967. 01730260106015.

Green, A.H. (1968) Self-destructive behavior in physically abused schizophrenic children. *Archives of General Psychiatry*. 19, 171-179. doi: 10.1001/archpsyc.1968.01740080043008.

Greenwald, B., Marin, D., & Silverman, S. (1986). Serotoninergic treatment of screaming and banging in dementia. *The Lancet*, 328, 1464-1465. doi: 10.1016/S0140-6736(86)92779-0.

Hajjar, R. R., & Kamel, H. K. (2004). Sexuality in the Nursing Home, Part 2: Managing Abnormal Behavior - Legal and Ethical Issues. *Journal of the American Medical Directors Association*, 5, 49-52.

Howell, T., & Watts, D. T. (1990). Behavioral Complications of Dementia: A Clinical Approach for the General Internist. *Journal of General Internal Medicine*, 5, 431-437. doi: 10.1007/BF02599434.

Johnson, C., Knight, C., & Alderman, N. (2006). Challenges associated with the definition and assessment of inappropriate sexual behavior amongst individuals with an acquired neurological impairment. *Brain Injury*, 20, 687-693. doi: 10.1080/02699050600744137.

Knight, C. et al. (2008). The St Andrews Sexual Behaviour Assessment (SASBA): development of a standardised recording instrument for the assessment and measurement of challenging sexual behaviour in people with progressive and acquired neurological impairment. *Neuropsychological Rehabilitation,* 18, 129-159. doi: 10.1080/09602010701822381.

Kuczynski, L., & Hildebrandt, N. (1997). Models of conformity and resistance in socialization theory. In J. E. Grusec, & L. Kuczynski (Eds.), *Parenting and children's internalization of values: A handbook of contemporary theory.* (pp. 227-256). Hoboken: Johen Wiley & Sons.

Kuczynski, L., & Kochanska, G. (1990). Development of children's noncompliance strategies from toddlerhood to age 5. *Developmental Psychology, 26* (3), 398-408. doi: 10.1037//0012-1649.26.3.398.

Kuhn, D. R., Greiner, D., & Arseneau, L. (1998). Addressing hypersexuality in Alzheimer's disease. *Journal of Gerontological Nursing,* 24, 44-50.

Lai, C. K., & Arthur, D. G. (2003). Wandering behaviour in people with dementia. *Journal of advanced nursing,* 44, 173-182. doi: 10.1046/j.1365-2648.2003.02781.x.

Lai, C. K. (1999). Vocally disruptive behaviors in people with cognitive impaitment: Current knowledge and future research directions. *American Journal of Alzheimer's Disease and Other Dementias,* 14, 172-180. doi: 10.1177/153331759901400304.

Luthra, A.S. (2013). *New Terminology to Label Behaviors in Dementias: Stage Congruent Responsive Behaviors (SCRB).* Manuscript submitted for publication.

Luthra, A.S. (2013). *Classification of behaviors in dementiabased in impairment in theories based upon information processing pathways.* Manuscript submitted for publication.

Luthra, A.S. (2013). *Classification of Behaviors in Dementia based in "motivational" and "needs based" theories.* Manuscript submitted for publication.

Luthra, A.S. (2013). *Classification of behaviors in Dementias based upon theories of regulation of emotions.* Manuscript submitted for publication.

Luthra, A.S. (2013). *Classification of behaviors in Dementias based upon principles of compliance and aggression.* Manuscript submitted for publication.

Magri, C.J., Ferry, P., Abela, S. (2007) A review of the etiology and management of vocal behavior in dementia. *Malta Medical Journal,* 19, 30-35.

Mahieu, L., & Gastmans, C. (2012). Sexuality in institutionalized elderly persons: a systematic review of argument-based ethics literature. *International Psychogeriatrics,* 24, 346 - 357. doi: 10.1017/S1041610211001542.

Masterman, D. (2003). Treatment of the neuropsychiatric symptoms in Alzheimer's disease. *Journal of the American Medical Directors Association,* 4, 146-154. doi: 10.1016/S1525-8610(04)70406-5.

Monteiro, I. M., Boksay, I., Auer, S. R., Torossian, C., Ferris, S. H., & Reisberg, B. (2001). Addition of a frequency-weighted score to the Behavioral Pathology in Alzheimer's Disease Rating Scale: the BEHAVE-AD-FW: methodology and reliability. *European psychiatry,* 16, 5-24.

Nagaratnam, N., & Gayagay Jr, G. (2002). Hypersexuality in nursing care facilities—a descriptive study. *Archives of gerontology and geriatrics, 35*(3), 195-203. doi: 10.1016/S0167-4943(02)00026-2.

Nagaratnam, N., Patel, I., & Whelan, C. (2003). Screaming, shrieking and muttering: the noise-makers amongst dementia patients. *Archives of gerontology and geriatrics*, 36, 247-258. doi: 10.1016/S0167-4943(02)00169-3.

Rheaume, C., & Mitty, E. (2008). Sexuality and intimacy in older adults. *Geriatric Nursing*, 29, 342-349. doi: 10.1016/j.gerinurse.2008.08.004.

Robinson, K. M. (2003). Understanding hypersexuality: a behavioral disorder of dementia. *Home Healthcare Nurse*, 21, 43-47. doi: 10.1192/apt.11.6.424.

Ryan, D.P., Tanish, SMM., Kolodny, V., Lendrum, B.L., Fisher, RH. (1988). Noise making amongst the elderly in long term care. *The Gerontologist, 28*(3), 369-371. doi: 10.1093/geront/28.3.369.

Stubbs, B. (2011). Displays of inappropriate sexual behaviour by patients with progressive cognitive impairment: the forgotten form of challenging behaviour? *Journal of Psychiatric and Ment Health Nursing*, 18, 602-607. doi: 10.1111/j.1365-2850.2011.01709.x.

Szasz, G. (1983). Sexual incidents in an extended care unit for aged men. *Journal of the American Geriatric Society*, 31, 407-411.

Teresi, J. A., Holmes, D., Dichter, E., Koren, M. J., Ramirez, M., & Fairchild, S. (1997). Prevalence of behavior disorder and disturbance to family and staff in a sample of adult day health care clients. *The Gerontologist, 37*(5), 629-639. doi: 10.1093/geront/37.5.629.

Tetlock, P. E. (1985). Accountability: A social check on the fundamental attribution error. *Social Psychology Quarterly*, 227-236.

Tucker, I. (2010). Management of inappropriate sexual behaviors in dementia: a literature review. *International Psychogeriatrics*, 22, 683-692. doi: 10.1017/S1041610210000189.

von Gunten, A., Alnawaqil, A. M., Abderhalden, C., Needham, I., & Schupbach, B. (2008). Vocally disruptive behavior in the elderly: a systematic review. *International Psychogeriatrics*, 20, 653-672. doi: 10.1017/S1041610208006728.

Wallace, M., & Safer, M. (2009). Hypersexuality among cognitively impaired older adults. *Geriatric Nursing*, 30, 230-237. doi: 10.1016/j.gerinurse.2008.09.001.

Chapter 9: Summary and Future Direction

To alleviate stress for the patient and care providers, expanding knowledge and creating evidence based treatment of BPSD has been identified to be a top priority for dementia/NCD research (Finkle et al., 1997; World Health Organization, 2012). To develop evidenced-based non-pharmacological and pharmacological treatments for any medical disorder, the profile of syndromes in that disorder must be identified. Attempts have been made to identify syndromal presentation of BPSD. Validated behavioral assessment scales utilized with this intent include Cohen-Mansfield Agitation Inventory (CMAI), Present Behavioral Scale (PBS), Behavioral Syndromes Scale of Dementia/NCDs (BSSD) and BEHAVE-AD (Robert et al., 2010).

Of these scales, the most frequently utilized is the BEHAVE-AD assessment scale (Conn & Thorpe, 2007). Each of the seven categories included in this BEHAVE-AD scale (delusions, hallucinations, activity, aggression, diurnal, affective, and anxieties) have been evaluated (Monteiro et al., 2001). In doing so, stable syndromes have been identified in aggressive behaviors (e.g., aggressive resistance, physical threats, active physical aggression, and verbal aggression); motor hyperactivity (e.g., walking more, aimless walking, moving objects, and trailing/shadowing); and depression (sad appearance, tears, and saying gloomy things). Additional work with the remaining scales also found aggression, depression and apathy to be reliable syndromes (Monteiro et al., 2001). Less reliable syndromes identified were motor hyper-reactivity and psychosis (Monteiro et al., 2001).

However, no syndromes were identified to be consistently occurring together when each of these behavioral categories was evaluated so as to collectively characterize a disease state or respond to a common pharmacological intervention (Robert et al., 2010). As an example, behavioral categories of "paranoid and delusional ideation", "activity disturbance", and "diurnal rhythm disturbance" have not been shown to fulfill the above in order to meet the criteria for a syndrome. Similarly, the behavioral category of "hallucinations", "affective disturbances", "activity disturbances", and "anxiety and phobias" have also failed diagnostic labeling as a syndrome. Likewise, no evidence could be found to support the presence of syndromes using the existing behavioral assessment scales (Robert et al., 2010). It is reasonable to deduce from the above data, either syndromes in dementia/NCD patients with BPSD do not exist or alternatively the existing behavioral scales lack the ability to detect the presence of such syndromes.

In the early stages of dementia/NCD it is possible to obtain a history from the patient and conduct a formal mental state examination with an appropriate physical examination and distinguish amongst different clinical states using established DSM-5 criteria. With advancing stages of cognitive impairment there is a decrease in reliability and validity of the history and mental state exam obtained from the patient. Under these conditions, greater emphasis is placed upon obtaining collateral information from all sources and on clinical observations, rather than clinical examination of the patient. Hence, it becomes difficult not only to identify a given clinical condition but also to distinguish amongst various clinical states or diagnosis (Cohen-Mansfield, 1997).

Herein lays the biggest challenge. How do you develop a behavioral assessment scale which maintains its reliability and validity in the absence of the patient's ability to participate in a valid clinical assessment; as is the case in all dementia/NCD patients with moderate to advances stages of cognitive impairment?

Hence, there is a need to develop a behavioral assessment scale which relies entirely on observations of the staff, family members, and specialized geriatric teams. Such a scale would be applicable to dementia/NCD patients in the moderate to advanced stages and who are unable to participate in a reliable and a valid clinical interview. The preceding chapters have identified 12 behavioral categories which have been constructed on the principles and constructs put forth by Davis et al (1997). These twelve (12) behavioral categories, with respective cluster of symptoms underneath each, have been formatted into an assessment tool titled "Luthra's Behavioral Assessment and Intervention Response" (LUBAIR) scale.

Disorganized Behaviors

- Appearing "vacant" or "blank" in facial expressions and mental lethargy
- Disorganized thinking, unintelligible/garbled speech
- Rapid shifts in or incongruence of emotional states
- Inappropriate mixing of food or clothing and layering smearing fecal matter, playing in the toilet bowl or global functional decline
- Playing with things in the air, responding to auditory hallucinations, picking things from the body or furniture
- Mental or physical lethargy or general functional decline

Misidentification Behaviors

- Misidentification of persons, places, objects
- Misidentification of sounds, smells, tastes or touch
- Misidentification of events or occurrences
- Misperception or interpretation of comments or behaviors of others

Goal Directed Behaviors (Cognitions and Activities)

- Goal directed cognitions such as, "I am going home today, I am going to the bank, I am getting married today, where can I pay my bills,"
- Goal directed activities (rummaging, rifling or emptying drawers; stripping clothes, rearranging furniture or fixing items in milieu; stripping bedding or pulling curtains/fixtures on the walls; bed/chair exiting or exit seeking; intrusiveness or purposeful wandering (seemingly driven, "on the go")

Vocal Behaviors

- Explosiveness, argumentative and quarrelsome
- Talking loud and fast, acting manic-like
- Whimpering, moaning, making strange noises, yelling and screaming
- Persistent calling out for staff/family or parents;
- Rattling bedrails, banging tabletops

Emotional Behaviors

- Appearing sad, despondent or tearful
- Expression of despair, morbidity, gloominess and helplessness
- Mimicking or mocking and being dismissive
- Sarcastic or Teasing, derogatory comments, being critical and negative of others
- Feeling rejected or increased sensitivity to comments from others

Fretful/Trepidated Behaviors

- Fearful or scared facial expressions
- Anxious or distressed facial expressions
- Clingy or "latches on", ringing of hands, rubbing face or body
- Expressing worry, fear, foreboding or catastrophe

Importuning Behaviors

- Persistently seeking reassurance or asking for assistance
- Behaving in ways for demands to be met immediately
- Shadowing staff
- Attention seeking or manipulative behaviors

Apathy Behaviors

- Indifference and lack of concern re: self and environment
- Lack of self-initiation, low social engagement (inter-personal interactions; and milieu structure) and poor persistence

- Emotional indifference and acknowledgement of lack of emotional remorse

Oppositional Behaviors

- Negotiating around care and other needs
- Working against everything the care giver or care provider is attempting with the patient
- Evasive to directions
- Resistive to care, medication or meals or other care directions;
- Barricading and territorialism

Physically Aggressive Behaviors

- Pulling, pushing, grabbing
- Kicking, biting, scratching, punching
- Spitting, throwing things, breaking objects
- Self-abusive/mutilating behaviors

Sexual Behaviors

- Verbally sexual (comments, gestures, innuendos)
- Physically sexual (grabbing breasts, buttocks, crotch)
- Self-stimulation (masturbating)

Motor Behaviors

- Roaming, strolling wandering
- Fidgety, rocking in wheelchair, restless, agitated;
- Seemingly driven, "on the go", wheelchair propelling, chair/bed exiting

Evidence based pharmacological interventions are available for the early stages of dementia/NCD. In the recently released DSM-5, the official classification of dementia/NCD is "major neurocognitive disorder" (NCG). In this book, both terms have been used. Cognitive enhancers slow down the progression of the disease, preserve functions and delay the emergence of neuropsychiatric and neurobehavioral sequelae. As long as the patient is able to engage in a valid clinical interview, provide a reliable history and participate in a mental status examination, clinical disorders can be determined using DSM-5 criteria. Such is the case in early to mild stages of dementia/NCD. However, as the reliability and validity of the information obtained from the patient interview diminishes, as is the case in moderate to advanced stages of dementia/NCD, it becomes difficult to determine specific co-morbid psychiatric disorders using DSM-5 criteria.

Behavioral and Psychological Symptoms of Dementia/NCD (BPSD) (equivalent to "behavioral symptoms of neurocognitive disorder" in DSM-5) is a diagnosis of exclusion. All separate and discrete mood, anxiety, & psychotic disorders, delirium, and all co-morbid psychiatric disorders have to be excluded in order to rule in BPSD. With the progression of dementia/NCD into moderate to severe stages, the reliability and validity of information obtained from the patient is severely compromised. There is increasing reliance for information on collateral sources and observational data. Furthermore, it is in the moderate to advanced stages of dementia/NCD the prevalence of BPSD is the highest; reaching up to 90%.

Several standardized scales have been used to distinguish amongst different co-morbid psychiatric syndromes in patients with moderate to advanced stages of dementia/NCD. Examples of these include Confusion Assessment Methodology (CAM) scale, Cornell Depression Scale and Neuro Psychiatric Inventory (NPI). Review of the literature clearly identifies that none of the above scales have an established validity and reliability in patients with moderate to advanced stages of dementia/NCD. Furthermore, all of these scales depend upon the patient to engage in a reliable and valid clinical interview to diagnose psychiatric co-morbidity; this is not reliable patients in moderate to advanced stages of dementia/NCD.

There are no currently available clinical tools available whose reliability and validity has been established for severely ill dementia/NCD patients. As a consequence, specific clustering of individual clinical symptoms are yet to be identified which are either consistent along temporal timelines or respond to a common therapeutic intervention. Attempts have been made to discern syndromes using standardized behavioral scales such as BEHAVE-AD. Whereas several clusters of symptoms have been identified, they have failed to respond to a common therapeutic intervention.

As a consequence, minimal progress has been made in developing overall effective pharmacological and affordable non-pharmacological interventions in the management of BPSD. There is evidence to support a small set of individual symptoms of BPSD responding to pharmacological treatments. However, the risks to the patient from the use of medications often outweigh its benefits. For these reasons, all best practice guidelines only recommend the use of medications sparingly and typically for a short duration. The use of non-pharmacological interventions as first line is more consistent with the first principle of medicine; *primum non nocere* (do no harm). Consequently, non-pharmacological interventions are considered the "gold standard," first line intervention for managing BPSD. The evidence for non-pharmacological interventions is not robust and they are extremely expensive to sustain. Furthermore, the skill set and training required to successfully implement non-pharmacological treatment is not readily translatable into every day clinical practice and the cost of implementing such a level is may be cost-prohibitive.

The incidence and prevalence of dementia/NCD is on the rise in the westernized world and is in keeping with the inverse pyramid of population demographics. The financial burden of caring for dementia/NCD will increase exponentially over the next three to four decades as the large cohort of baby boomers ages. Hence, to have minimally effective pharmacological treatment and rather expensive and un-sustainable non-pharmacological treatment for management of BPSD is simply an unacceptable state of clinical affairs, especially when up to 90% of the patients who go on to develop dementia/NCD will exhibit BPSD. We are yet to fathom the consequences of the "White Tsunami".

One way forward is to make an effort to understand the *"meaning"* for the presence of behaviors in patients with dementia/NCD. Understanding the *"meaning"* of behaviors is an essential step in order to make substantive progress in the management of BPSD, with pharmacological and non-pharmacological interventions, in dementia/NCD care. With this goal, guidance was sought from existing published literature for developing novel approach to labeling and classifying behaviors in moderate to advanced stage of dementia/NCD in order to better understand the *"meaning"* of these behaviors.

After an extensive review of the existing literature and identification of obvious deficiencies, a new theoretical framework for labeling behaviors in patients with dementia/NCD has been proposed. The newly proposed model and terminology provides an alternative to the existing models which are dichotomized along the biological and psychological paradigm. This new model is a comprehensive biopsychosocial (BPS) model for understanding of the occurrence of behaviors in dementia/NCD. Review of literature identified multifaceted factors contributory to the occurrence of behaviors in patients with dementia/NCD. Biological factors (stage of the disease, presence or absence of co-morbid psychiatric illness, inherent circadian rhythms and innate physiological needs), personal factors (pre-morbid personality and acquired coping strategies) and environmental factors (milieu structures and interpersonal interactions) were all identified as playing a significant role in the generation of behaviors in patients with dementia/NCD. A complex interplay amongst each of these variables was posited to justify the generation of a comprehensive BPS *model* and the appointment of new *terminology* to label behaviors in dementia/NCD: *Stage Congruent Responsive Behaviors (SRCB) (pronounced "scrub").*

Subsequent chapters in the book have focused on the development of a new theoretical framework for classification of this newly appointed *terminology* to label BPSD. Criteria put forth by Davis et al (1997) were identified as the most appropriate principles as the basis of classification of the newly developed terminology of SCRB.

- Review of the literature was done to identify various "specification of the theoretical constructs" to justify the aggregation of similar behavioral symptoms into clinically meaningful categories.
- Each of these behavioral categories represents a specific purpose to the patient exhibiting them and portrays a meaning of their presence to the care givers and care providers.
- Such a paradigm to a consistent understanding of the meaning for the presence of behaviors in patients with moderate to advanced stages of dementia/NCD is a land mark step in assessment and management of these behaviors.

From the existing literature, the following theoretical constructs were identified as the "specification of the construct" for each behavioral category developed:

- Behaviors based in Information Processing Theories

- Behaviors based in Motivational and Needs Based Theories
- Behaviors based in Theories on Regulation of Emotions
- Behaviors based in Theories on Principles of Compliance and Aggression
- Heterogeneous group which encompasses behavioral categories requiring a combination of the above theories

Two behavioral categories emanating from pathological changes in *Theories of Information Processing (TIP)* are described:

Disorganized Behaviors (DOB)

DOB is the result of an alteration in the physiological status of the patient from baseline. Such an altered physiological status results in changes in arousal and attentiveness, collectively known as the sensorium. Changes in the sensorium result in impairment of the sequential organization of information processing thereby giving way to fragmentation of the process at many different levels of the brain. This results in impairment in generation of cognitions, emotions and behaviors.

MisIdentification Behaviors (MiB)

MiB are the result of a specific breakdown in two specific steps in information processing: schema identification and pattern recognition. This results in the failure of the usual pairing of old and new information; an essential step which provides context in processing of new information. Absence of this contextual pairing of information results in an altered sense of relatedness between self and persons, places, objects and events. This leads to misidentification of visual, auditory, tactile, gustatory and olfactory perceptions and content and behaviors of others.

Four behavioral categories emanating from pathological changes in *Theories of Motivation* and *Needs Based Theories* are described. A discrepancy between a patient's internal and external environment leads to identification of a need. Adequate motivational forces are required to propel the individual in order to statiate these needs. Apathy Behaviors (AB), Goal Directed Behaviors (GDB) and Motor Behaviors (MB) are the consequence of pathology in theories of motivation. Importuning Behaviors (IB) are the result of preserved motivational drive and the specific need being identified and fulfilled through expression of these behaviors are the basic "physiological' needs.

Apathy Behaviors (AB)

- AB is the consequence of a decrease in motivational drives which results in absence of fulfilment of all needs identified by the individual.

Goal Directed Behaviors (GDB)

- GDB are the result of an increase in the motivational drives due to disease states. The specific need requiring fulfilment is the "belongingness" need. There is an increase in the detection and fulfilment of these "belongingness" needs due to disease states.

Motor Behaviors (MB)

- MB is the result of varying degrees of changes in motivational drives. MB is the most non-specific of all BPSD and, in themselves, do not portray any message other than an indication of a state of unrest in the patient. MB is often a concomitant with any of the other behavioral categories identified.

Importuning Behaviors (IB)

- IB is the result of preserved motivational drives in dementia/NCD patients. The specific need being identified and fulfilled through expression of these behaviors are the basic "physiological' needs.

Three (3) behavioral categories emanating from pathology in *Theories of Regulation of Emotions.*

Emotional Behaviors (EB)

- EB are based in the expression of two of the primary emotions of "melancholy" and "discontentment". EB based in primary emotion of 'melancholy" is primarily allowing the patient with a measured catharsis of emotional pain. This leads to a state of decompression from emotional pain and re-establishing a state of emotional homeostasis. EB based in the primary emotion of discontentment serve a protective purpose for the patient. These behaviors often tend to break down all lines of communication between the patient and their milieu. This pre-emptive effort is designed to make the patient less vulnerable to emotional hurt from others. This is like building a wall of around one's ego as a protection mechanism.

Fretful/Trepidated Behaviors (FTB)

- FTB are based in expression of the primary emotion of fear. The specific need requiring fulfilment in these patients is the 'security' need. The presence of these behaviors signifies an inadequate fulfilment of security needs. These behaviors highlight the pathological attachment models in the index patient expressing these behaviors.

Vocal Behaviors (VB)

- No singular specific theoretical construct could account for the heterogeneity of symptoms found in these behavioral categories. It has required every single specification of theoretical construct identified to account for various sub-types of VB and SB identified in this new classification.

Sub-types of VB identified are

1. VB (aggressive type)
2. VB (effusive type)
3. VB based in GDC
4. VB based FTB and/or IB
5. VB based in self stimulation (SS)

Two behavioral categories emanating from pathology in *Theories of Compliance* and *Theories on Aggression*.

Oppositional Behaviors (OB)

- In accordance with theories of compliance, there is a bidirectional dynamic relationship between the patient and their milieu. The patient attempts to preserve this state of homeostasis. The emergence of OB is the direct consequence of non-compliance by the patient to directions from caregiver or care providers. The subtypes of OB emerging are determined by the level of developmental sophistication of the patient, the degree of cognitive impairment in the patient and a very dynamic impact of the latter on the former variable.

Physically Aggressive Behaviors (PAB)

- PAB are an expression by the patient of a perceived impediment in goal attainment. The expression of PAB is to make the caregiver or provider aware of the relationship between the origins of negative emotions, such as anger and discontentment, as a consequence of blockage in goal attainments. Acts of physical aggression are a sum total of continuation of direct defiance to persistent directions to an out of proportion emotional responses accompanied with functional motor activities. Physical aggression can also be the sum total of continuation of direct defiance to persistent direction and perceived impediment to goal attainment of not wanting to change the existing state of homeostasis.

Likewise, no singular specific theoretical construct could account for the heterogeneity of symptoms found in Sexual Behaviors (SB). SB have also required every single specification of theoretical construct identified to account for various sub-types SB identified. Sub-types of SB identified are

1. SB based in Misplace Intimacy (MI)
2. SB based in Attribution Error (AE)
3. SB based in Stimulus Bound behaviors (SBB)
4. SB based in Importuning (IB)
5. SB based in Innate need for Intimacy (INI).

Future Direction

Dementia/NCD Care is a fast emerging clinical subspecialty in medicine which cuts across several of the established clinical specialties and inclusive of Geriatric Psychiatry, Geriatric Medicine, Behavioral Neurology and even Primary Care practice in Long Term Care and institutional settings involved in the care of the elderly. In my opinion, dementia/NCD care is a "spring board" specialty where professionals from any of the above aforementioned specialties can gain added training to practice in it. The text book is focused on furthering the knowledge base in the area of dementia/NCD care.

The ultimate goal of this new theoretical constructs and clinical paradigm is to develop effective and safe pharmacological treatments and more sustainable and affordable non-pharmacological treatments to manage behaviors in patients with moderate to advanced stages of dementia/NCD. Optimal treatment for all medical disorders always involves the best balance of pharmacological and non-pharmacological interventions.

The approach to assessing behaviors in patients with dementia also requires redefining terms for the following reasons;

a) Terms 'acute' and 'chronic' are qualifiers for time lines of onset and progression of a disease, including those for behaviors in dementia (American Psychiatric Association, 2000). In context of behaviors in patients with dementia, 'acute' refers to emergence of behaviors in patients in whom none were present. 'Chronic' refers to the presence of behaviors for a prolonged duration of time but only came to the recent attention of the health care professionals once a specific risk has been identified. The latter appears to be the most commonly occurring reason for referral of dementia patients with behaviors in long term care facilities.

b) No specific distinction has been made in published literature between the approaches to assessing 'acute' and chronic' behaviors in patients with dementia. It would appear both terms have been used inter-changeably for all clinical and research purposes in this patient population.

Clinical guidelines are in existence for assessment of 'behaviors' in dementia though no distinction is made between the approach to 'acute' onset and 'chronic' behaviors. The approach to assessing 'acute' and 'chronic' behaviors is as follows;

a) Identify 'reversible' or 'modifiable' variables likely contributory.

b) Second step is to view the presence of behaviors as a consequence of a perturbance in the homeostasis between the demented patient and their environment. This paradigm to labelling behaviors is captured using the antecedents-behaviors-consequences (ABC) approach (Davis & Luthans, 1980).

It is a commonly occurring situation where all medical investigations have failed to identify an identifiable etiology and no specific environmental triggers are recognized. Yet, the behaviors remain, as is the case in the vast majority of dementia patients with chronic behaviors. There is an absence of direction from published literature in the approach to assessing these chronic behaviors with regards to the following issues:

a)   Are all behaviors present of clinical significance?
b)   How should the clinical significance of behaviors be defined?
c)   How should the severity of the clinically significant behaviors be defined?
d)   What is the best way forward in developing a uniform approach to addressing the aforementioned issues and thereby decreasing the vast inter-clinician variability in the approach to assessing and managing behaviors?

Preliminary steps undertaken to accomplish the aforementioned goal are:

Each of the behavioral categories identified were used to develop a new behavioral assessment tool titled: Luthra's Behavioral Assessment and Intervention Response (LuBAIR) Scale. A proposal was submitted to the Research Ethics Board at McMaster University, Hamilton, Canada to conduct validation and reliability study on this new behavioral tool. LuBAIR Scale was compared against Cohen-Mansfield Agitation Inventory and Behave-AD scale. The permission was granted and the study has been undertaken. Results have been tabulated and manuscript is being prepared for submission for publication to a peer reviewed journal.

Development of a Clinical Handbook on utilization of LuBAIR scale in clinical practice. The clinical handbook has been written and will be submitted for publication after the acceptance of the reliability and validation study on LuBAIR to a peer reviewed journal. Clinical Handbook will provide clinicians with a new theoretical framework to define Quality, Frequency, Duration and Severity of behaviors thereby providing a uniform approach to their assessment. Clinical Handbook will further provide constructs to define risks associated with each quality of behavior identified through the use of LuBAIR scale.

Identification of each quality of behavior, which is represented in the LuBAIR scale as each individual clinically meaningful category, has the potential of identifying specific syndromes in patients with dementia of various etiologies and through different stages of the disease. It is being hypothesized that:

- The behaviors occur as a 'constellation of behavioral categories' i.e. a syndrome, in each individual patient.
- For a dementia/NCD patient, of any given etiology, these syndromes are unique to that patient at each specific stage of their disease. The staging of the disease is mild, moderate, severe and advanced and in accordance with MMSE scores.
- Hence, the syndromal presentation in the mild, moderate, severe and advanced stages of the disease are different for that individual with any given etiology.
- Identification of stage of disease specific syndromes should give us better direction in developing affordable non-pharmacological and judicious pharmacological treatment intervention in a systematic manner

A research proposal was submitted to Research Ethic Board at Homewood Health Center, McMaster University to evaluate these hypotheses. The meaning of the behaviors derived from each behavioral category was also used to develop non-pharmacological interventions for patients admitted to Dementia Care Unit (Hamilton 3), Homewood Health Center, Guelph, Ontario. Furthermore, the new classification systems used to develop LUBAIR have been used to develop pharmacological treatment algorithms in the management of behavioral risks. The results are being evaluated. Preliminary data is extremely encouraging whereby the behaviors have been managed successfully without the loss of cognition or function as a side effect from the use of medications.

This text book is specifically targeted towards Geriatric Psychiatric specialists, Geriatric Medicine specialists, Neurologists and post-graduated Behavioral Psychologist and Gerontology health care professionals. In addition to targeting the aforementioned health care professionals this book can also be targeted towards Family Doctors in Geriatric primary care, Clinical Nurse Specialists and all Registered Nursing and allied health care staff (Occupational Therapists, Social Workers, Physiotherapists and Speech language Pathologists) working in Dementia/NCD Care.

www.ingramcontent.com/pod-product-compliance
Lightning Source LLC
Chambersburg PA
CBHW060320220326
41598CB00027B/4378